The Powerwatch Handbook

Simple ways to make you and your family safer

Alasdair and Jean Philips

PIATKUS

Copyright © 2006 by Alasdair and Jean Philips
First published in Great Britain in 2006 by
Piatkus Books Ltd
5 Windmill Street, London W1T 2JA
email: info@piatkus.co.uk

The moral right of the authors has been asserted

A catalogue record for this book is available from the British Library

ISBN 0 7499 2686 4

Text design by Richard Mason
Edited by Barbara Kiser

This book has been printed on paper manufactured
with respect for the environment using wood from
managed sustainable resources

Typeset by Palimpsest Book Production Limited,
Polmont, Stirlingshire

Printed and bound in Great Britain by
MPG Books, Bodmin, Cornwall

Dedication

This book is dedicated to Eddie and Marion, who have made enormous improvements to the lives of so many people.

About CHILDREN with LEUKAEMIA

The authors' royalties from the sale of this book are being donated to the CHILDREN with LEUKAEMIA Charity.

In February 1987, leukaemia killed Paul O'Gorman at the age of 14 years. CHILDREN with LEUKAEMIA was established the following year in fulfilment of the promise that Paul elicited from his parents – to help other children with leukaemia. It is now Britain's leading charity dedicated to the conquest of childhood leukaemia.

Leukaemia is a complex disease and we know little about what causes it. The incidence rate of childhood leukaemia increased steadily during the last century. This strongly suggests that there is something about our modern way of life which is increasing the risk of leukaemia in our children. A variety of factors have been linked with childhood leukaemia, including exposure to electric and magnetic fields, air pollution and radiation as well as the pattern of exposure to infectious disease in childhood. Such influences may exert their effect at different stages – in the womb, after birth, or even before conception.

A link between childhood leukaemia and electricity was first revealed in 1979. Three decades on, the evidence continues to strengthen but we still don't understand the underlying mechanisms. CHILDREN with LEUKAEMIA is the main charity funding research into the various causes of childhood leukaemia, including electricity.

Contents

Acknowledgements

Sarah, Ruth, Graham, Simon & Amy have been more tolerant than we could hope for. Our friends have supported us when we have neglected them. Those who know us and love us have been there in our chaotic lives more than we have any right to wish for. For this words can not express our gratitude, but thanks anyway.

There have been so many people guiding our footsteps along the uneasy path we have chosen to tread. We can only mention a few, or the list would be longer than the book.

If in error, and in a senior moment or two, we have omitted your name, you will know who you are and this is for you, too.

To Ross Adey, Neil Cherry, Louis Slesin, Roger Coghill, and especially Denis Henshaw, thanks for having been there, to share the midnight oil teasing out the difficult questions.

To Ray & Denise, Anne & Eddie and all the wonderful parents and children we have visited, we owe you more than we can express. Thanks for the cups of tea and the invitations to share the joys and sorrows of your lives.

To Simon Best, Maureen Asbury, Eileen O'Connor and friends, the world would be a more hazardous place without your unstinting efforts. We value your friendships more than you probably realise.

To the team at Piatkus and above all, Helen, thanks for your unending patience, without your prodding and encouragement this book would never have reached the light of day. Thanks for that.

To everybody who has tried the tips we have suggested and have reported back their experiences, this book is as much yours as ours.

Long may you all remain as healthy as possible.

Alasdair & Jean

Foreword

We live in a world in which convenience is the raison d'être of progress. Microwaves, mobile phones, MP3 players, laptops, you name it, the race for comfort and accessibility is being won, a victory evidenced by the plethora of electrical goods on the market. We now live in a world that few sci-fi enthusiasts could have foreseen. And I love it. I love the ease and speed at which I can retrieve information, listen to music, contact people, heat my food, and lead a full life. It is a world that I am sure you have come to love as well; one we are so used to, so in love with, that the very idea that such convenience may carry health risks, is almost tantamount to a betrayal of what it is to be modern.

But we must face this possibility. These much loved electrical goods produce electromagnetic fields (EMFs) that swirl around us invisibly everyday, wrapping us in vibrating electrical frequencies that are far higher than those naturally emitted by the earth. But what are we to make of this? Does it matter? Do we really have anything to worry about? Well this book maps out an excellent path to the answers.

And it could not come at a more timely point. Public unease shows no sign of subsiding over mobile phone masts despite government assurances. Vested industry interests and government reluctance to really engage in a debate about EMFs, all mean that there is no clear guidance as to what to do about them. Few lay people know what they are, what they do and if or why they should be worried about them.

I am all for more research in this area. As a former scientist I am always on the hunt for truth, the smoking gun, something definitive. But as the authors so aptly note, science today is complex, smoking guns are rare and as such the hunt for a definitive truth has morphed into a puzzle of probabilities.

As the scientists, politicians, public health officials and others attempt to decipher the puzzle, it is imperative for us to become more active, to take a bit more responsibility for our own health and that of our families. That is why I am such a fan of this book. It is a refreshing jargon-free handbook that aids understanding and gives helpful, pragmatic tips. Happy reading.

Dr Ian Gibson, MP
Former chair of the UK House of Commons
Science & Technology Committee

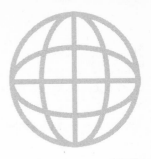

Introduction

It is amazing to think that a century ago, the man-made energy that surrounds us now didn't exist. The Italian-born scientist, Marconi, had just managed to send the first radio signal across the Atlantic. It wasn't until 1920 that the Marconi Company began the first public speech transmissions from Chelmsford in the UK, when Britain, despite being one of the first countries to introduce electrification in residential areas, was still largely electricity-free.

Now, in the 21st century, we live in a world utterly changed. And it is all down to electrification. Our homes are filled with labour-saving devices, entertainment to suit every taste and information at the touch of a button, while public and private transport are faster and safer than ever before.

You can now control lighting and heating with a switch or knob or even by a microchip sensing your presence in a room. You can buy automatic-flush toilets, microwave ovens – and very soon, freezers designed to read the codes on your food and send this information to a shopping list on your computer using microwave signals to let you know what items in your freezer need replenishing. You can surf the web with broad-band. You can talk to people any time, from anywhere, using your mobile phone or internet connection.

Yet despite these luxuries, inconceivable to our Victorian pred-ecessors, many of us find ourselves more stressed and under the weather than ever before.

Opting for a high-tech lifestyle means that we have all become surrounded by 'electrosmog' – a sea of electric and magnetic fields (EMFs) from powerlines, house wiring and appliances, radio, TV, mobile phone and mast signals, and other microwave sources. In fact, since the start of the 20th century, our exposure to man-made EMFs has risen to a point where we are now experiencing levels literally millions of times higher than anyone living in Marconi's time.

As a result, all of us have become guinea pigs in a great elec-tromagnetic experiment.

We believe that electrosmog is the cause of some of our stress, and that it may be responsible for serious health prob-lems for you and your family. And it is for people like you that we have written this book.

You may simply have heard about electromagnetic fields and want to find out more. You may have found that the World Health Organization is monitoring research into EMFs. Or you may have encountered some of the many articles reporting on possible links between disease and EMFs – such as leukaemia 'hotspots'.

Below are a number of these stories. They do not amount to conclusive evidence, but they are a cause for concern and within the context of the available scientific evidence, which

we've gathered in the scientific appendix to this book, we feel
they are also a call for action.

Power trouble

In March 2001, an article appeared in the *Sunday Times*. It
was about the Smith family, who have lived for three decades
in a North Yorkshire house that lies in the shadow of an electricity pylon. The family had no history of cancer. But in 1996,
the mother died of cancer, and the father now has the
disease. A son died of liver cancer, aged 18, in 1988. The
family cat and dog, along with a neighbour's pet, have all been
diagnosed with cancer. Janette, the Smiths' daughter, is
convinced that the powerlines have triggered the cancers.

The Smiths' story is tragic, but by no means unique. In the
same area, for instance, the secretary of the local branch of
the National Farmers' Union found nine cases of cancer in 19
houses along a five-mile stretch of powerlines. And there are
many more such cases, all over the UK.

In Abergavenny, in Wales, 4 neighbours living near
powerlines developed brain tumours over a period of
18 months.

In the 8 houses closest to powerlines in Kilmarnock,
Scotland, 9 people have died of cancer over the last
15 years.

In Dalmally, also in Scotland, in a small estate of 36
houses under a 275,000-volt powerline, 8 people
died of cancer in 5 years, and 3 of motor neurone
disease (MND).

A street in Exeter, Devon, where a 132,000-volt electricity pylon looms outside the homes of some of the residents, has been dubbed 'Death Road'. In 28 houses, 23 people have died from heart disease or cancer. In fact, the number of cancer deaths on the road is five times higher than the norm for Devon and Cornwall. Residents also complain of depression, headaches and memory loss.

Also in Devon, a seven-year-old girl called Emma who lived near a 15-metre-high mobile phone mast was diagnosed with leukaemia. The mast beamed right through Emma's house to reach the town centre. Emma's mother was then diagnosed with breast cancer, and another three residents in line with the mast also developed cancer. After extensive local protests and national media coverage, Orange finally agreed to move the mast to a more suitable location.

The *Birmingham Post* reported in 2004 that people living in the Midlands village of Wishaw, near Sutton Coldfield believe a mobile phone mast is to blame for their health problems, which include cancer. Almost eighty per cent of people living near a mast at Wishaw, near Sutton Coldfield, have become ill: five with breast cancer, one with prostate cancer and one with lung cancer, three with pre-cancerous cervical cells, and one with MND – a man who has also had a massive tumour removed from the top of his spine. Some of the villagers have developed benign tumours, and some have reported they are suffering from electrical hypersensitivity. In November 2005, the 70-foot mast at Wishaw was torn down by a person unknown. Since then, the health of many of the local residents has been gradually improving, and a number of previously infertile women are now in the later stages of pregnancy. Fearful of a new mast being erected, they blockaded the site for months, preventing T-Mobile from putting up new equipment.

In 2002, people in a village in County Tyrone, Ireland, blamed a nearby mast for an 'epidemic' of cancers. John Thomson, one of the stars of the TV series *Cold Feet*, was reported as saying he and other local residents were 'sick with worry' about the potential health problems when a mobile phone mast was due to be built nearby. His partner was expecting a baby at the time. 'If the government has said these masts shouldn't be built near schools, how can it be all right to have one so close to the home where we plan to raise our child?' asked Thomson.

In 1989, the Studholme family bought a bungalow in Greater Manchester. An electricity meter in a cupboard in the hallway emitted a strong electromagnetic field through the wall into the front bedroom. Their son Simon slept with his head less than a yard from this meter. He started to complain of pains, but the doctors found nothing wrong. Within 18 months he had developed acute lymphatic leukaemia. He died in 1992 at the age of 13. Subsequent tests revealed that Simon had been sleeping in an electromagnetic field of over 2.5 microtesla (a measurement of electromagnetic field strength), more than sixty times the average exposure level in UK homes. The UK Health Protection Agency guidance allows exposure up to 100 microtesla.

Acute and deadly diseases are not the only possible effects of EMFs. There are chronic problems, too. These are the result of sensitivity to EMFs, a condition known as electrosensitivity which we discuss fully in Chapter 8.

> Peter, a dental technician, needs bright illumination for his work, and has several fluorescent lights, some only 18 inches (45 cm) above his head in his small work-room. The room also contains other electrical appliances and some high-power tools. Peter suffers from a lot of painful physical symptoms, depression, anxiety, hallucinations and chronic fatigue. He has attempted suicide three times and has had six nervous break-downs. He loves cooking, but gets very stressed if he is near kitchen appliances for more than half an hour.
>
> Joe is also electrosensitive. He has had to move home three times in the last two years and has had to completely re-wire the house each time using screened mains cable. He can no longer drive or use public transport because of high EMFs from the vehicle and from passengers using their mobile phones.
>
> Betty's electrical sensitivity is increasing. Three years ago she could use a landline telephone and watch television. Today she feels unwell the moment she tries to use a telephone, and she cannot cope with more than an hour of television.

We have been studying such reports for more than 20 years, sifting and analysing the evidence and disseminating it through books and the media. Now, Powerwatch advises the UK government and is accepted as the foremost source of independent information about EMFs and health in the country. Here is our story.

How Powerwatch began

Alasdair Philips first began thinking about electromagnetic fields in the context of human health back in the early 1980s, when he was asked to help the women anti-nuclear war protestors camping outside the US Air Force base at Greenham Common in Berkshire, in the UK. The protestors claimed they were being 'zapped', and together with some friends in the group Electronics and Computing for Peace Alasdair discovered that their claims were true.

The protestors were being targeted with pulsed microwave radiation from prototype electromagnetic 'non-lethal' weapons then under development by the US military. Some of these were to be publicly acknowledged and demonstrated by the Pentagon starting in 2001.

After Greenham Common, Alasdair became aware that a much bigger public health issue was not being discussed – that of ordinary powerlines and electricity in the home increasing the risk of children developing cancer, especially leukaemia. For well over 20 years, the biggest influence on Alasdair by far has been Louis Slesin's writings in his regular news report, *Microwave News*. Slesin has been reporting, in a well-documented, fair and objective way, the potential health and environmental impacts of electromagnetic fields and electromagnetic radiation since 1981.

By 1989 it had become clear that there were questions being asked all over the world about the safety of EMFs.[1]

Some of the first warnings had come in 1972 when scientists in the Soviet Union reported strange health effects in switch-yard workers who were routinely exposed to high levels of elec-tromagnetic fields. The workers experienced increased heart disease, nervous disorders, blood pressure changes, recurring headaches, fatigue, stress and chronic depression.

Alasdair, an electronics engineer and scientist, joined forces with Neil Mayhew, a road safety engineer, to set up the independent organisation Powerwatch in the late 1980s. Jean has been helping him in his work since the 1990s. They began to assess the available research and, as far as possible, provide an independent view on the debate, without industry or government bias.

When the 1984 UK Telecommunications Act was passed, the revolution in personal wireless communications exploded on to the scene. All was believed to be well, until mobile phone users began to report health symptoms, primarily headaches and disorientation – and, with time, cancers of the brain and neck. Some of the early story was covered in *The Zapping of America* by Paul Brodeur in 1987.[2] The technical background to mobile phone and health issues was added to in Robert Kane's 2001 book and the 'insider's view' was controversially brought more up to date by George Carlo in the same year.[3] They showed that the industry was well aware, from the 1980s, of biological changes leading to possible adverse health problems and had been doing their best to suppress public awareness of this knowledge.

Since the work of Powerwatch was first mentioned in the UK national newspapers in 1988, it has been an active, well-respected voice promoting precaution with regard to human exposure to electromagnetic fields.

The *Stewart Report*

Public concern and unrest about mobile phones grew following the widespread international media publicity given to Roger

Coghill's court case, brought in November 1998 to require handsets to carry health warning labels. Coghill is one of the few independent scientists researching into links between EMFs and health. Alasdair was the main technical witness. As a result, in the summer of 1999 the UK health minister instructed the National Radiological Protection Board (now the Health Protection Agency's Radiation Protection Division) to set up a completely independent committee to examine the science behind mobile phone safety. Known as the Independent Expert Group on Mobile Phones (IEGMP), the committee was chaired by Sir William Stewart. Sir William, a consultant medical doctor, was the UK Chief Scientific Adviser, Cabinet Office, 1990–1995.

Powerwatch was invited to contribute both written and oral evidence for consideration by the expert group. Stewart expressed his surprise when representatives of campaign groups invited to present their experiences to the committee were more worried about mobile phone *base stations* than the phones themselves. The committee report, made public in May 2000 and known as the *Stewart Report*,[4] recommends to the government 'that in making decisions about the siting of base stations, planning authorities should have the power to ensure that the RF (radio frequency) fields to which the public will be exposed will be kept to the lowest practical levels that will be commensurate with the telecommunications system operating effectively.'

This was not done. In January 2005 Stewart's update re-affirms: 'The Board believes that the main conclusions reached in the *Stewart Report* in 2000 still apply today and that a precautionary approach to the use of mobile phone technologies should continue to be adopted.'[5]

The *Stewart Report* is not the only high-level document to find potential links between EMFs and human health.

The California study

In 2002, California's Department of Health Services published a £4.5 million, nine-year study on EMFs for the state commission on public utilities – the biggest such report so far.[6] The three epidemiologists who authored the report concluded that raised levels of EMFs increased the risk of cancer, particularly childhood leukaemia, miscarriages, adult brain cancer, and ALS, a form of progressive motor neurone disease also known as Lou Gehrig's disease.

The levels of EMFs studied by the California team can be found not only near powerlines, but also near household appliances. This Californian study did not look at the sort of pulsing radio-frequency/microwave emissions that can be found near mobile phones and masts, but there is increasing evidence that these result in the same sort of health problems (see the Appendix).

Leading edge – Powerwatch now

Throughout the rise in public concern over these issues, Powerwatch has played a vital role in presenting well-argued precautionary advice in the public domain.

The group is seen as a key member of the government's Stakeholder Advisory Group on mains electricity EMFs (SAGE), which is helping to formulate recommendations for government policy on powerfrequency EMF precautionary advice and guidance.[7]

Over the last 12 years, Powerwatch has published several books (see Further Reading) which include research on how the health problems linked to EMFs could be explained, in terms of both traditional and cutting-edge biology, biochemistry, neuropsychoimmunology, physics and electronics.

Alasdair has also spoken at, and chaired, many international conferences. We are frequently interviewed as the UK's leading independent source of information on EMF concerns for television documentaries such as *Panorama*, national and local news programmes, television journals such as *Countryfile* and radio investigations like *Costing the Earth*. We are often asked to comment on these issues in research and news stories, national and local newspapers, magazines and journals.

An ongoing debate

The subject of electromagnetic fields and possible health effects generates debate and high emotions. Whenever a news story appears, there are always disagreements between different scientists, campaign groups, government and industry spokespeople as to what all the information means.

Trying to understand the complex interrelationships involved is not an easy task and few people have expertise in all the areas involved. After all, only a small percentage of adults have studied physics, electronics, biology or chemistry at university level; and many didn't even study them at school. And those who did study one of these sciences – whether they now work in the field or not – often have little knowledge of the others. For instance, very few physicists or engineers are knowledge-able about neurophysiology and the biological sciences, and hardly any biologists have any significant grasp of pulsing elec-tromagnetic signals and how they may interact with life. Even those who have been taught biophysics at university have usually learned the old paradigm of electromagnetic fields – 'if it doesn't heat you, or electrocute you, it doesn't hurt you'. We now know that this is wrong.

So not just the general public, but the science community –

and the government committees, campaign groups and industries the scientists seek to inform – may not see the whole picture when it comes to EMFs and human health. And, indeed, the jury is still out on a number of the possible effects.

But at Powerwatch we feel it is vital to share what we know so far. And, most importantly, we want to advise you on how you can protect yourself and your loved ones from the known and the suspected risks.

At Powerwatch, we believe the evidence for these risks is getting stronger. We believe that the electrosmog surrounding us all is getting more 'aggressive', and also more difficult to avoid. And that's where this user-friendly handbook comes into its own. It will fully inform you of the problems, so you can choose to take action, where appropriate, to protect yourselves from adverse health effects – while still taking advantage of some of the benefits advanced technology offers.

How to use this book

The Powerwatch Handbook will prove invaluable when you find you:

- need to buy an electrical appliance
- are thinking of buying or renting a home
- want to rewire your house
- see electrical installations, such as powerlines or substations, near where you live and wonder if your home may be affected
- see an application for a mobile phone mast near where you live
- wonder whether you may be affected by EMFs at work
- are deciding how to travel somewhere

- read about a new technological 'gadget'
- want to have a child
- want to protect your children, yet also want them to have access to 'safe' modern technology
- want to find out about your own, your children's or grand-children's new electronic plaything
- want to furnish a new nursery
- want to check your child's nursery or school
- want to avoid becoming electrically sensitive
- want to find out about some of the EMF research findings – the reality behind the issues.

We have written *The Powerwatch Handbook* so that you can choose the safest *type* of product you want. If there is a wide range of options, you may decide to measure the EMFs to make your final selection. Powerwatch has developed a range of easy-to-use instruments to measure the EMFs (see EMFields in Resources) and make this process as easy as possible. By buying or hiring these instruments, you can compare the fields you are exposed to with the levels which have been shown by international research to be associated with an increased risk of serious health problems. This gives you the information you need to be confident you are making the right decision to help protect you and your family from the hazardous effects of living with some modern technology.

Note that we don't discuss EMF levels of manufacturers' particular models, but only particular types of appliances or gadgets. The reason for this is that manufacturers often make several different models of a particular type of appliance, and in EMF terms some will be better than others. The models themselves change far too rapidly to keep track and such details would quickly be out of date, and therefore misleading.

Using the symbols

Chapters 3 to 7 in the book discuss particular items of electrical equipment in common use, such as telephones, cookers, computers, TVs and the like. To help you select the safest item we have developed a coding system to indicate whether a particular type of appliance is likely to radiate high EMFs (powerfrequency or radiofrequency), and whether some types are better than others.

☺ The more happy faces there are, the lower the EMFs. The lower the EMFs, the less likely it is that you will react.

🗑 The more bins there are, the higher the EMFs. The higher the EMFs, the more likely it is that you, someone in your family, or someone you know may be affected.

If you are interested in finding out more about Powerwatch and our campaign for a safer world, please see our website (see Resources for details). We hope that all of you will find this book interesting and helpful, and will join us in trying to make the world a safer place

Alasdair and Jean

1

EMFs and Our Health

In this chapter, we'll be looking carefully at EMFs and their effect on our health. We believe that there is now plenty of evidence that continuous exposure to electromagnetic fields in our living environment can sometimes cause serious ill-health effects. Most authorities are now signing up to a more precautionary approach to possible environmental hazards than was the case in the past. This is sometimes expressed as the 'precautionary principle', which recommends taking reasonable actions to reduce possible harm to the environment and our health where there is a suggestion of possible harm but scientists have not yet found 'proof of harm'.

The debate centres around what is 'reasonable'. This can range from just making the public aware of a possible problem, to fixing warning labels on products and even changing codes of working practice. A good example is the 'low EMF radiation' computer monitor (VDU). Initially requested by Swedish trade unions, the idea was dismissed by the computer industry as unnecessary and too costly ('it will double the price'). However, Nokia saw a market niche and went ahead and produced some

VDUs that did cost considerably more than the standard product. These were sold to governments and major companies. Within a few years almost all manufacturers were making similar models and competition meant that the cost of low emission VDUs soon fell below the cost of the earlier high EMF models!

Deciding what is reasonable in terms of our health is not usually an easy process. Who can you turn to for the answers? When you remember the controversies about smoking, passive smoking, HIV & Aids, asbestos, BSE and global warming, it is easy to see how we can all end up feeling very confused about serious issues that affect us and our children. However, we ignore them at our peril. These issues have important implications for our own health, and the health and sustainability of the planet.

Although we would all prefer it if safety issues were 'somebody else's problem', leaving the complicated issues to scientists and 'experts' is no answer, as we know that vested interests play a significant part in the telling of 'truth'. Different groups, organisations and individuals want different things.

- The government wants a thriving economy, a quiet life, free trade in a competitive market and popularity.
- Business wants a thriving economy with maximal profits and no onerous duties or liabilities.
- Scientists want interesting problems and continued research funding. They have seen colleagues who 'have rocked the boat' ending up with severe funding problems and many now shy away from politically contentious areas of research.
- Pragmatists, like Powerwatch, and the insurance industry want a 'fair balance'.
- Most of us want the benefits of modern ways of living without endangering our health.

To make the best informed decisions, we need to be aware of these different agendas, and to accept that it is our responsibility, as individuals, to ensure the safety of our personal environment. We at Powerwatch help in this process not just by disseminating the findings of sound research, but also by revealing the factors that can cloud the issues and even affect scientific outcomes. We look at some of these at the end of this chapter. (For the scientific evidence for, and discussion of, EMF effects on human health, see the Appendix on page 234.)

Now let's get to grips with the EMF-health connection. In order to understand it, we start with a closer look at EMFs themselves.

All about EMFs

EMFs are produced as a result of the flow of electric current from the power station, where electricity is produced, to the places where we wish to use it. EMFs can be measured surrounding the power cables hanging between electricity pylons, near substations and near cables, both overhead and underground. The wiring in our houses, the electric appliances and lights we use, all produce EMFs.

At mains-frequency, the magnetic fields and the electric fields need to be considered separately, and there are different safety guidelines for each. At high frequencies, such as those used for telecommunications, magnetic and electric fields are so linked they are usually considered together as 'electromagnetic radiation'. Microwaves, X-rays, radio waves and light are also electromagnetic waves. ('Frequency' means the number of vibrations per second, so 'high frequency' means more vibrations per second.)

In our homes we are surrounded by EMFs; from the house wiring and from the appliances which use the electricity supply. The three illustrations below show examples of EMFs in the home.

Switched off

This picture shows *electric* fields from sockets and from the wire to the lamp, even though the light is not switched on.

These electric fields are present all the time electricity is present in the wires, even if it is not actually being used.

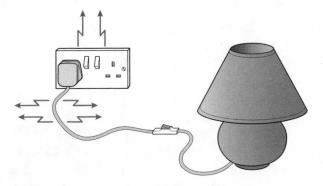

Electric Fields

Switched on

The second picture shows the electric and magnetic fields from the lamp when it *is* switched on. The electric fields now extend to the lamp. *Magnetic* fields are also being produced by the current flowing along the wire and light bulb – although these usually reduce quickly as you get further away.

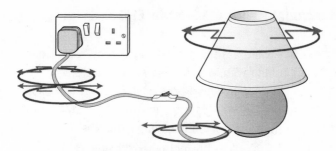

Electric and Magnetic Fields

At the socket

The following illustration shows a common type of mains-adapter transformer that converts the 230 volts mains electricity to a lower voltage needed for many, usually portable, electronic devices. Once again, both electric and magnetic fields are emitted. The magnetic fields are considerable and can still be high up to half a metre away from the transformer. Sometimes transformers are built into radios and music players and are actively emitting magnetic fields all the time the player is plugged into the mains, even when it is not actually in use.

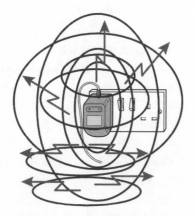

Electric and Magnetic Fields from plug transformer
(mains adapter)

The trouble with man-made EMFs

In the pre-electric era there were only natural electromagnetic fields to contend with, and these were not a problem. For instance, the geomagnetic field – which causes compass needles to point north – is a natural source of EMFs emanating from the Earth's magnetic core. It is a fairly steady background magnetic field and does not vibrate each second. Because we have evolved with it, it is generally safe for us.

However, there are problems with man-made EMFs. EMFs from mains electricity vibrate at 50 to 60 hertz (Hz) – which means that the electromagnetic signal constantly repeats itself 50 to 60 times per second. This phenomenon is new to our environment. It's known that constant physical vibration is generally not good for the health of people or animals, and we believe that this constant electrical 'vibration' has negative health effects.

There is a fairly steady electric field between the Earth's surface and the sky of about 100 volts per metre (V/m) in good weather. Natural vibrations in this field above 1 hertz are tiny (less than one-hundredth of a volt per metre). This is very different to the changes in field levels near electrical wiring and equipment, where the 50/60 Hz vibrations can be very much greater (several hundreds of volts per metre), 'shaking' our cells in ways that many scientists believe can have a detrimental effect on our health.

As we saw in the introduction to this book, since the start of the 20th century we have been gradually exposed to more and stronger EMFs as more and more gadgets and equipment using electricity and radio waves have appeared.

We are now surrounded by electric and magnetic fields millions of times stronger than those we experienced a mere century ago. As long ago as 1991 the *US National Regulatory Research Institute Bulletin* said: 'Public concern over the risk to health of electromagnetic fields is likely to become one of the most important environmental public health issues.'

One alarming development in this context is the rise of EMFs at microwave frequencies. Microwaves – which are very high-frequency and used not just in microwave ovens, but also for mobile and cordless telephones, video and data transmission and other home, work and school equipment – are rare in nature. But since the Second World War, we have managed to boost the amount of microwave energy surrounding us many millions of times. Modern communications systems transmit this energy in a pulsed way that we believe can adversely affect your health.

Safety standards – are they adequate?

The official international guidelines on EMF safety set by ICNIRP – the International Commission for Non-Ionising Radiation Protection – do not in any way acknowledge that cancer and the other health effects covered in this handbook are associated with electromagnetic field exposure. For instance, the 50 Hz magnetic field guidance level for the general public is 250 times higher than the exposure level that is now accepted internationally as being associated with a doubling in incidence of childhood leukaemia.

We believe that, as a precautionary measure, *magnetic* field levels in bedrooms and other places where people spend a lot of their time should be less than 0.1 microtesla and *electric* fields less than 15 volts per metre.

As laid down by ICNIRP, safe levels for the general public are only to protect people against heating and electric shock. At mobile phone frequencies, ICNIRP allow microwave signal levels 1,200 times greater than those being reported by medical doctors as causing such adverse health effects as headaches, sleep problems, blood pressure problems and depression. You will find more on all this in later chapters.

Some occupational studies looking at the health of workers exposed to EMFs have found disturbing evidence that levels well below the guidelines are associated with a significant rise in leukaemias and other diseases such as amyotrophic lateral sclerosis or ALS, a form of motor neurone disease.

High-frequency EMFs, radio frequency, and especially microwave radiation, have also been linked to serious health problems since radiofrequency energy has been used. Safety guidelines were drawn up to protect people exposed to this form of radiation at work from heating effects. There is increasing evidence that long-term exposure to pulsing microwaves at much lower levels can have implications for health.

In the next chapters we will be discussing specific EMF sources. There is evidence that a number of illnesses are triggered by, or associated with, EMF exposure from these sources, but the disease that has so far been most closely connected to EMFs is childhood leukaemia.

The link with childhood leukaemia

The strongest evidence that EMF exposure adversely affects human health can be found in studies done on EMFs and childhood leukaemia. Nancy Wertheimer, an American biologist and experimental psychologist, was the first to discover this link.

A trail in Colorado

In 1974, after some 20 years spent raising her family, Wertheimer decided to get back to public health work. She was interested in the idea that childhood leukaemia, a disease virtually unknown before the 1920s, might have an environmental cause.

Even though she had no funding, Wertheimer decided to carry out an exploratory investigation, looking for any sort of observable pattern. From the Colorado Department of Vital Statistics she obtained a list of the home address at birth of every child in the Greater Denver area who had died of leukaemia between 1950 and 1969, along with birth addresses of matched children without cancer. (Note that it would be almost impossible to get this kind of information for research purposes nowadays.)

Armed with these addresses, Wertheimer drove round the city, stopping at every house on the list and noting down environmental details. She did not come across any unusual cluster of cases, though she kept seeing electricity poles with black cylindrical transformers mounted on them and numbers of feed wires to nearby houses and apartments. These transformers are like very small electricity substations, changing the 13,000 volt supply down to 120 volts – the normal voltage supply for American homes.

She found that the cases of childhood leukaemia were usually in one of the three homes nearest to the transformer. 'I was puzzled, but thought it must be a fluke,' she later told the *New Yorker* magazine.

Wertheimer then contacted an old physicist friend, Ed Leeper, to see if he could think of any likely electrical effect. In

December 1974, Ed built a simple but sensitive magnetic field meter that also indicated the strength of the field by the loudness of a hum given off by a small loudspeaker.

When they revisited the homes near the transformers, they found very loud buzzing near the poles, indicating high levels of 60 Hz magnetic fields. In the autumn of 1975, Leeper built Wertheimer a meter that could accurately measure the magnetic fields. Wertheimer spent most of the next 18 months, still in her own time and unpaid, travelling around the Denver area taking magnetic field readings and noting other possible factors such as population density, air pollution and traffic noise.

The two spent much of the next year working with the data and writing what was to turn out to be a landmark paper that put EMFs firmly on the international cancer research agenda. It was published in the *American Journal of Epidemiology*'s March 1979 issue as 'Electrical Wiring Configurations and Childhood Cancer'.[8]

The picture now

In order to discover whether the finding by Wertheimer and Leeper revealed a real problem or was a fluke, much of the subsequent research into the effects of EMFs concentrated on powerfrequency magnetic fields and childhood leukaemia. It has now been accepted internationally, even by the most cautious of organisations, that living in EMF levels above 0.4 microtesla will double the risk of your child developing this form of cancer before the age of 15 – from about 1 in 1,600 to 1 in 800.

This acceptance is based on two meta-analyses of many high-quality international studies. Yet despite all this evidence, there is little enthusiasm among governments for announcing precautionary measures to limit EMF exposure. One sign of hope, however, was the formation of the Stakeholder Advisory Group on EMF in 2004. SAGE, which is jointly funded by the Department of Health, National Grid Transco and CHILDREN with LEUKAEMIA, advises the UK government on the issue of precautionary EMF advice and is expected to report before the end of 2007.[9]

Meanwhile, despite enormous improvements in treatment and survival rates, leukaemia remains the most common cancer in children under the age of 15. In the UK, about 500 children are diagnosed each year and about 100 die from it.

The incidence of leukaemia and some other childhood cancers in developed nations has been rising at around 1 to 3 per cent per year for the past 50 years. The graph below shows this trend for the UK. As childhood leukaemia was almost always fatal before 1960, data on deaths was used where data on diagnosed cases was not available. There is no officially recognised cause for this rise, although possible reasons are being explored – for instance, at the 2004 CHILDREN with LEUKAEMIA international scientific conference in London.[10]

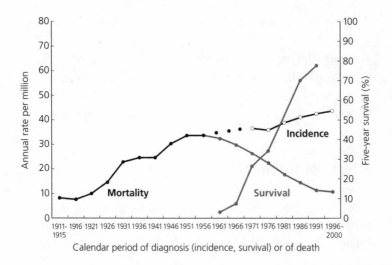

Calendar period of diagnosis (incidence, survival) or of death

Worryingly, this kind of leukaemia is now also on the rise in countries developing a Western-type lifestyle. Studies led by Dr Sam Milham in the US show that the rise in childhood leukaemia followed the electrification of the different states. A peak in leukaemia in children two to four years old emerged in the UK in the 1920s, and slightly later in the US. Milham and his colleague E M Ossiander concluded that this peak is due to electrification.[11] In 1920, half the urban and rural homes in the US that were not on farms had electricity, compared to 1.6 per cent of farm homes. Electrification in US rural and farm areas lagged behind urban areas until 1956 and enabled them to investigate the progression. Their study clearly shows the rise of the 2- to 4-year-old childhood leukaemia peak from 1920 to 1960. Something new was happening that was affecting the health of American children, which Milham and Ossiander blamed on the arrival of electricity.

EMFs and other serious illnesses

A number of other diseases and conditions have been associated with EMF exposure, among them adult cancers including brain tumours, clinical depression and suicide, miscarriages, Alzheimer's disease and other dementias. (See the Appendix)

A strong EMF link has been shown with amyotrophic lateral sclerosis or ALS, known as Lou Gehrig's disease, a fatal form of motor neurone disease that develops in late middle age.[12] At any one time there are about 4,500 cases in the UK and 30,000 cases in the US.

Effects of mobile phones

Since about 1985 the use of mobile phone technology has expanded from the odd few people experimenting with business phone accessibility when travelling, to the present day when you are considered to be very unusual if you do not have and use a mobile phone. Many homes no longer have landline telephones, but only mobile or digital cordless (DECT) phones, which use the same technology as mobile phones. If you have one, you have effectively installed the equivalent of a small mobile phone mast right inside your home or office.

Developing countries are opting for mobile phone systems rather than a wired system as the cable network for a wired phone is more expensive than a network of masts.

Some evidence points to cancers and other serious health problems arising from exposure to mobile phone and phone mast radiation. We look at specific conditions linked to phones, and safety precautions, in Chapter 3, and masts are discussed in Chapter 2.

We look at some of the relevant science in the Appendix.

Effects of light at night

Light is just another part of the electromagnetic spectrum, lying between microwaves and X-rays. Reliable evidence is building up that we all need a regular light/dark cycle every 24 hours to be healthy.[13]

But these days, night is becoming almost as light as day over much of the Western world, and increasingly in the developing world. Photographs from space of parts of the Earth at night reveal a network of light, with bright patches over urban areas and road networks.

Much of the research into the effects of exposure to light at night has focused on the pineal gland. Located in the centre of the brain, this gland produces the hormone melatonin when it is dark.

Among the most important of the tasks melatonin does in the body is repairing normal, day-to-day cellular damage. Damage to cells can trigger cancer. People who work at night under lights and thus never experience a period of relative darkness have a higher rate of cancer than people who work during the day. People with impaired sight (whose eyes and/or brains do not register light in the same way) have a lower rate of cancer than sighted people. Melatonin is also involved in mood control, and people with clinical depression have often been found to have lower levels of this hormone.

For more on light and our health, see Chapters 4 and 7.

Electrical hypersensitivity – the new syndrome

We undeniably live in a polluted world, and in the process of living in it, our bodies can become sensitised to environmental stresses. As a result we may find we react badly to certain chemicals, develop food intolerances, or begin to suffer from asthma or eczema.

You can also develop sensitivity to the presence of EMFs. This condition, known variously as electrosensitivity, electromagnetic hypersensitivity, or electrical sensitivity or hypersensitivity, can have very serious consequences not just for your health, but for the way you live your life. In essence, electrical hypersensitivity or EHS – the term we use in this handbook – has become part of the increasing problem of environmental stress.

EHS is a reasonably new syndrome, significantly affecting probably 3 to 5 per cent of the population of industrialised societies – a number that in England alone represents nearly 2.5 million people. Perhaps up to 35 per cent of people show some indications of electro-stress.

Many of the symptoms people with EHS report also show up in other stress-related conditions, which makes it difficult for EHS to be accepted as an independent diagnosis.

If you have EHS, you will typically experience a number of symptoms that appear or get worse near electrical appliances (computer monitors are commonly a problem), powerlines, fluorescent lights, mobile phones, mobile phone base stations and/or other EMF sources, and diminish (or occasionally disappear) the further away from the EMF source you are.

To discover whether you have, or might have, EHS, complete the questionnaire below. The list of symptoms is based on the November 2005 report *Definition, Epidemiology and Management of Electrical Sensitivity* by Neil Irvine, for the Radiation Protection Division of the UK Health Protection Agency. Most people will experience some of the symptoms listed for reasons which have nothing to do with EMF exposure. However, the higher your score, the more likely it is that you have EHS.

Do you suffer from electrical hypersensitivity?

Score as follows:
If you have the symptom described
Frequently, score 2
Occasionally, 1
Never, score 0

Do you suffer from:
1. Numbness, weakness or prickling sensations in your joints or limbs
2. Feelings of abnormal tiredness or weakness that cannot be explained by your life commitments

3. Changes in your ability to think clearly or finding it difficult to concentrate, depending on where you are
4. Aches and pains, cramps or muscle spasms in your joints, bones and muscles in your shoulders, arms, legs, feet, wrists, ankles, elbows and pelvis. Fibromyalgia
5. Headaches
6. Tenseness
7. Restlessness, anxiety
8. Memory loss
9. Sleep disturbance, insomnia
10. Feebleness, dizziness, tremors
11. A tendency to skin redness, itchiness, rashes, tingling or dry skin
12. Abdominal pain, digestive problems, irregular bowel movements, sickness
13. Feeling too hot, fever
14. A smarting, irritating sensation, a pain, or a feeling as if there is grit in your eyes. Blurred vision or flickering before the eyes
15. Nosebleeds or blood pressure changes
16. Heart arrhythmias or irregularities, palpitations or chest pain
17. Toothache or neuralgia
18. Hair loss
19. Hearing clicks, humming, buzzing, hissing or a high-pitched whine
20. Sensitivity to light, especially fluorescent lights or computer screens (sometimes, though rarer, even daylight)
21. Bouts of unusual irritability, rage, violence, destructiveness, feeling hostile
22. Thyroid problems
23. A generalised feeling of impending influenza that never quite breaks out
24. Depression
25. 'Missing time', blackouts or convulsions.

If you scored 15 to 25 out of 50, you may be one of the 35 per cent of people suffering from some degree of electro-stress. If you scored more than 25, you may have developed EHS.

For more information on avoiding or minimising EHS, see Chapter 8.

So far, we've seen that the evidence for EMFs being harmful to health is accumulating, although general agreement regarding their negative effects centres on childhood leukaemia. In looking at the evidence, we at Powerwatch feel it is vital to remember that there are a number of factors affecting how research is done that can in turn have an impact on outcomes. We give some examples below.

Who can you trust?

The influence of industry

One of the central problems in science today is the intrusion of vested interests. Much research relies in part on funding from industry, and while the vast majority of scientists simply want to explore areas of interest, they often need to follow the money. They may also shy away from politically contentious areas of research because they've seen how 'rocking the boat' can lead to withdrawal of funding.

United Nations agencies are regarded as top authorities in their fields, but even they are not exempt from this intrusion. The World Health Organization (WHO) is vital to any discussion of EMFs because in 1996 they established the International EMF Project to assess the scientific evidence for possible health effects of EMFs. And yet the WHO has regularly obtained staff 'on loan' from industry and from universities where they have industry-funded posts. Many members of the EMF project itself have a long-standing industry bias.[14] For more information visit the Powerwatch website at www.powerwatch.org.uk.

On top of this, experiments are often designed so that the results are likely to be in industry's favour. When the results of a particular piece of research show that there is an industrial pollution-related health problem, it is disappointing just how often the researchers lose their funding. A case in point is the work of Denis Henshaw.

In 1999, Professor Denis Henshaw and his colleagues at Bristol University in the UK first revealed a scientific mechanism regarding how adverse health effects could occur near to high-voltage powerlines.[15] This received considerable media publicity around the world, and assessors at the Medical Research Council (MRC), which funded the research, viewed it as important. The company owning most of the powerlines wrote a strong letter of complaint about the publicity to the vice-chancellor of the university.

When Henshaw's MRC grant came up for renewal a few years later, it was refused 'due to a shortage of money'. There is no proof that his failure to receive a new five-year programme grant was related in any way to his outspoken stance about a controversial issue; but he was unable to continue the research until the charity CHILDREN with LEUKAEMIA stepped in with a new grant.

Standing agreements

Sometimes, it's not directly industry that may be affecting the course of research; it's related organisations. One of the best-known cases of this is the agreement between the WHO and its fellow UN agency, the International Atomic Energy Agency (IAEA).

Signed in 1959, this agreement effectively vetoes WHO research into the effects of radiation. The IAEA was set up by the UN in the 1950s to promote the development of nuclear power. The WHO is committed to attaining the best possible health for all peoples. Given the known health effects of ionising radiation emitted by radioactive sources like nuclear waste, this is an odd alliance. And after the Chernobyl nuclear accident of 1986, when large areas of the Ukraine, Belarus and Russia were badly contaminated, it affected science reportage in a problematic way.

Cancer rates in Belarus, for instance, were reported in the November 2004 *Swiss Medical Weekly* as rising by 40 per cent between 1990 and 2000 – that is, 6,000 *extra* deaths from cancer a year. This is only one such finding among many. Yet in September 2005 the Chernobyl Forum, a group of eight UN agencies including WHO and the IAEA, issued a 600-page report, *Chernobyl's Legacy: Health, Environmental and Socio-Economic Impacts*, stating that by mid-2005 fewer than 50 deaths have been directly attributed to radiation from the disaster.

Some eminent scientists, mainly with connections to the nuclear industry, were unconvinced that radiation was the cause of the 90-fold increase in rates of thyroid cancer in Belarus, arguing publicly that the radiation levels were too low to cause cancer. However, in May 2005, Elizabeth Cardis and

35 colleagues of the International Agency for Research on Cancer (IARC) announced a strong correlation between the radiation dose children received and their risk of developing thyroid cancer.[16]

In cases like this, just who should we believe?

Obstacles to inquiry

Whether or not something affects us, positively or negatively, depends on how we are – physically, mentally and emotionally – at the time of exposure, and what else we are being exposed to, including EMFs.

The results of laboratory work, where animals with short life-spans are tested under controlled conditions, do not constitute a conclusive test. The only way to assess something like the effects of EMFs is by carefully monitoring the effects of the environment and lifestyle on the health of real people living in the real world – the science of epidemiology.

This kind of research is not just difficult in itself; it is also hampered by the fact that in most countries, because of the right to privacy, it is becoming almost impossible to carry out good epidemiological work. The late Sir Richard Doll, the eminent epidemiologist whose discoveries include the link between smoking and lung cancer and between radiation and leukaemia, said in the August 2002 edition of *Epidemiology*:

> There has been an enormous change in the attitude towards confidentiality. I wouldn't say that it was a change in the public attitude, so much as in the govern-mental attitude, because I am not sure that the public is really as concerned as governments appear to be. When I started in epidemiology, we operated on the old system,

which was approved by the Medical Research Council, that a doctor could pass information about a patient to another doctor, relying on the fact that he or she would be bound by the Hippocratic oath to treat details about patients confidentially. We had no difficulty in collecting all sorts of information as long as the process was covered by someone medically qualified. Now it is becoming horrifyingly difficult to get hold of epidemiological information relating to individuals, and I can see great difficulties for the epidemiologists of the future. I find it so depressing, as valuable research of importance to the public health really is being made extremely difficult, if not impossible in some cases.

Sir Julian Peto – who holds the Cancer Research UK Chair of Epidemiology at the Institute of Cancer Research and the London School of Hygiene and Tropical Medicine – echoed Doll's words when he wrote in the *British Medical Journal* in 2004:

The deaths that will occur because of the effects of data protection law on British medical research attract less publicity than child murders; but the pointless obstacles that bona-fide researchers, particularly epidemiologists, face when they seek access to individual medical records are now causing serious damage.

At Powerwatch, we too have come across this problem when trying to organise EMF-related research on cancer. It is virtually impossible to get cancer data that includes people's postcodes – not their name and address, which are obviously not needed. Full postcodes are key in helping to identify clusters of cases where some environmental toxic agent such as radiation may have been implicated.

There are other factors that affect research into environmental triggers for illness, particularly cancers. A central one is the long timescale involved from the inception of the disease to full-blown cancer – this can take many years.

It is difficult to build up a clear picture of EMFs' effect on our health. While the evidence is growing, we recommend you take precautionary measures in your own lives in order to protect yourself and your family. The practical information that follows is our view based on our work and experience over the last two decades. Let's begin with a look at EMFs in the outside environment.

EMFs in the Outside Environment

If you commute or simply do a lot of travelling for whatever reason, you'll see and be exposed to a staggering array of EMF sources in towns, in cities and in the countryside. Everywhere you look there are powerlines, electricity substations, cables, electric railways and tramways, radio and television broadcast aerials, mobile phone masts, and airport, coastguard and military radar units and security systems.

Sources of EMFs are an ever-increasing feature of our environment. But this is not a cause for panic. We want to make it clear that in and of themselves, there are no 'good' or 'bad' sources of EMFs. In fact, many of them are necessary to maintain our 21st century lifestyle. The important factor is how many and what new types of transmitters are irradiating the environment.

We believe that the key thing here is that you spend as much time as possible in fields as low as can be achieved – and as little time in high fields as possible.

Just passing by EMF sources is unlikely to affect your or your family's health unless any of you are electrically hypersensitive

(EHS). However, we recommend that you start to become aware of the presence of these sources, and avoid them where this doesn't cause too much disruption in your day-to-day life. And, if you're thinking of moving house, we recommend that you take account of all the sources in the area you'd like to move into.

The level of EMFs is almost impossible to predict in practice, so we always advise people to measure them. (You can hire or buy instruments that will measure EMFs from EMFields – see the Resources section for details.)

Our safety ratings

In places where we discuss EMF exposure when, for example, you are travelling, we use a single ☺ or 🗑 to indicate whether there is likely to be a problem. Where extra care is recommended, we have used 🗑 🗑 .

Powerlines

Powerlines have been crossing rural landscapes and threading their way through cities for decades now to bring us the electricity we want to keep home, work, shops, gyms, cinemas, theatres, hospitals, clinics and schools running. You would not want to be without electric power, so it is important to have the information you need to be able to live with it safely.

Types of powerline

Powerlines are very visible EMF sources and come in a number of shapes and sizes. The largest are, of course, the massive cables strung between large metal 'transmission towers' or pylons.

In the UK, these carry 400,000 volts (400 kilovolt, or kV). The next largest are 275 kV. Both these types of powerline and the towers are owned and controlled by National Grid Transco. These are the lines that carry electricity from power stations to local distribution points, usually located outside main towns and cities.

At distribution points, the voltage is transformed down to 132 kV and below. These lower voltage lines, going eventually right down to 230 volts to power your home, are owned and maintained by the 10 regional UK energy network companies.

Once the voltage is transformed to 33 kV, 11 kV or lower it is usually carried on wooden poles. In rural areas, if they are overhead, you will see the local 400 and 230 volt lines carrying power to your home strung on wooden telegraph-type poles. The lower the voltage, the more likely it is that the cables will have been buried underground. (See below for a discussion of underground and overground lines.)

Underground vs overhead cables

In the countryside, all the 11 kV lines and above are usually overhead. In most urban areas all lines up to 33 kV are underground. In large towns, lines up to 132 kV are usually buried, but there are many places where these pass right over the roofs of houses. In cities, and a few special places, lines up to 400 kV may be underground.

Many powerlines have to cover a large distance from the power station to the cities, towns and villages where the electricity is to be used. They may cross particularly beautiful areas of the countryside. When new powerlines are being planned or upgraded, particularly through this kind of landscape, there is often a lively debate over whether the cables should be laid underground.

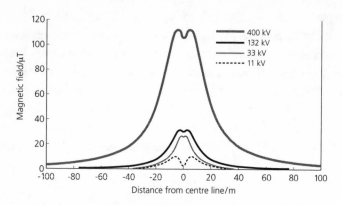

Maximum magnetic fields from overhead powerlines

The graph shows the maximum magnetic fields likely to be experienced when you are near to high voltage overhead powerlines. Typical levels are lower than these.[17] We believe that the 'safe' residential level is less than 0.4 µT, right down near the bottom line of the graph.

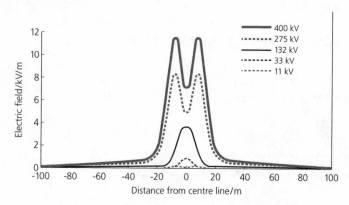

Maximum electric fields from overhead powerlines

The graph shows the maximum electric fields likely to be experienced when you are near to high voltage overhead powerlines.[18] We believe that the 'safe' residential level is less than 10 V/m, right down near the bottom line of the graph. Note the left-hand axis is scaled in kV/m (1000s of V/m).

Aesthetics are not the only thing improved by burying cables. Underground lines are more reliable in the long term, and the electric fields they emit are absorbed by the earth above them, making them safer to a degree.

But they do tend to cost more. The Energy Networks Association (ENA) – which represents the UK's licensed gas and electricity transmission and distribution companies – says that underground powerlines usually cost between 10 and 20 times as much to install as high-voltage overhead lines. At 11 kV and lower volt-ages, the cost will only be a few times more than the cost of an overhead line and the buried lines, as well as being more reliable are also cheaper to maintain. The cost of burying 400 kV lines can be between £10 million and £25 million per kilometre. The ENA says that any additional costs incurred as a result of changing to underground lines would have to be borne by the consumer.

All new estates are being built with underground cables. Given the advantages, we agree with this move, and also believe electricity companies should be encouraged to bury existing lines. The main concern with respect to underground cables is with their magnetic fields, which, unlike the electric fields, are not absorbed by the surrounding soil.

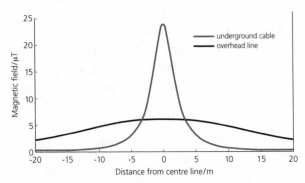

Comparison of typical magnetic fields from 400 kV overhead and underground powerlines

The graph shows a comparison of the typical magnetic fields likely to be experienced when you are near to an overhead or an underground high voltage 400 kV powerline. Note that although the fields are much higher directly above the underground line, they fall off much more quickly and are fine by about 20 metres (compared with over 100 metres for the overhead line).

EMFs round powerlines

So much for the kind of powerlines you may find in your immediate vicinity and on your travels – now let's look at the EMFs they emit.

In a high-voltage powerline, electric current flows along the cables. This creates:

- **Electric fields** from the **voltage** – that is, the electrical pressure that exists between the wires and the ground
- **Magnetic fields** caused by the **power flow** along the wires.

The electric and magnetic fields do not radiate from the metal pylons, as these are insulated from electricity. The most powerful fields are close to the lines themselves. When you move away from a line, your degree of exposure lessens. How far away you need to be to reach any 'safe' level depends on the voltage of the line (for the electric field) and the power it is supplying (for the magnetic field).

Generally speaking, the higher the voltage, or power, the further away you have to be for the EMF levels to be reduced significantly. Possible exceptions to this are the fairly common 132 kV lines, where you may have to be further away than you would expect for the EMF levels to be within safe limits. For magnetic fields, about which the evidence is the strongest, we recommend that the ambient background level is below 0.2 microtesla. Childhood leukaemia incidence is seen to be doubled at 0.4 microtesla, therefore 0.2 microtesla adds an extra safety margin for your protection.

EMFs from powerlines

As a very approximate rule of thumb, EMFs are likely to drop to below the 0.2 microtesla level at about:

- 150 metres from 400 kV lines
- 120 metres from 275 kV lines
- 100 metres from 132 kV lines
- 50 metres from 66 kV lines
- 30 metres from 33 kV lines
- 15 metres from 11 kV lines
- Closer with respect to local 415/230 volt lines.

The magnetic field levels vary considerably with the power the line is carrying at the time. The *only* way to know for certain what the EMF levels are, is to measure them.

Often the load carried by these 132 kV lines is unbalanced – that is, different currents go down the set of cables on one side of the towers compared with the other. When this happens, the magnetic fields do not cancel so well and the levels will be higher, and you'll need to be further away to reach the safety level.

National Grid Transco have connected up almost all of the 275 kV and 400 kV lines in a special way known as 'reverse phased', which minimises the strength of the magnetic fields you will be exposed to. However, few of the 132 kV lines operated by the regional companies have been connected like this. The only way for you to get a reliable idea of the field from powerlines is to measure them with a meter. It is almost impossible to estimate the levels because of the many variables involved. For example, while the maximum magnetic field level under many 400 kV lines will normally be less than about 5 microtesla, sometimes the fields can be 10 times higher than this.

If, using a meter, you do not get a magnetic field or electric field reading under the powerline, it is likely that it has been decommissioned temporarily or permanently. Check with National Grid Transco or the local electricity company to find out when it is due to restart, and measure the fields then. If the lines are no longer in use, the company has an obligation to remove them.

Our recommendations

Underground cables

☺ We believe that a safer option for electricity distribution is a system of underground cables. Each cable should effectively occupy a 'corridor', and housing should only be built starting at its outer boundaries, where the magnetic field levels have dropped to an acceptable precautionary level. (Assuming the cables are properly laid, the surrounding soil would, as we've mentioned, absorb the electric field.) There would be no problems associated with pollutants attracted to overhead cables, either (see below). We feel the benefits to health outweigh the financial costs.

🗑 **Magnetic fields** are a distinct problem with underground cables. These fields travel through almost anything. When you stand on an underground cable, you will be exposed to much higher magnetic fields than when standing under an overhead cable, because you are closer, but the fields fall off much faster with increasing distance.

Most cables are laid in shallow trenches (0.6 to 1.8 metres deep) and covered by soil, pavement or road surface. If there is a cable buried under the pavement in front of a house where there is a very small front garden or none at all, the fields in the room(s) at the front of the house, especially on the ground floor, could be high.

Basement flats in cities can also be exposed to strong magnetic fields from the cables running under the pavement outside.

In a few places, high power cables have been run in deep tunnels which alleviates the problem and reduces human exposure to the fields, but it is a very expensive technique and can only be afforded in special circumstances.

Overhead cables

🗑 Live cables going directly over a house or flat will almost certainly emit a magnetic field at a strength that has been associated with an increased risk of serious ill health. This can often be seen in villages and towns where the electricity supply runs through overhead cables, and a house has little or no front garden, leaving the poles relatively close to the house.

With this kind of scenario, magnetic field levels inside bedrooms can be high.

☺ In some rural areas the houses are supplied by overhead low-voltage (230 volt) cables strung between wooden poles. Aerial bundled cable (ABC cable) which looks like one thick twisted cable, emits much lower levels of magnetic field than four individual wires, because the cables are run close together and twisted, which neutralises much of the field.

🗑 Work carried out by a team at Bristol University has shown that air pollution can be made more dangerous by high-voltage powerlines. The high electric fields and 'corona' discharge around the wires (arcing or sparking into the air from the wires and also around the insulators' wire attachment – a phenomenon sometimes visible as a blue glow in damp conditions at night) 'charge up' all sorts of airborne pollutant particles, including those associated with cancer. Charged particles are more dangerous because they are more likely to attach themselves to people, especially their skin and lungs.

Charged particles can be blown up to several kilometres away from powerlines. If you live in an area with a lot of industry, crop spraying or busy motorways, powerlines can increase the risk of health problems arising from the pollution produced. Exposure to the chemicals used in crop spraying has also been linked to the development of chemical sensitivity and EHS.

🗑 Pylons and visible powerlines affect **property values**. For instance, in wet weather, larger powerlines can be heard to hum or 'sizzle' with corona discharge and the sound can worry some people, although in itself it does not necessarily indicate an increased danger to people nearby.

More importantly, over the years there has been enough publicity about the risks for people to question whether their health may be affected by living close to a high-voltage power-line, and the association with an increased risk of childhood leukaemia is now well established. In fact, many if not most potential buyers are now more concerned about possible health effects than any visual impact made by pylons and powerlines. Houses are a big investment, and people will be far less willing to put money into something that may become devalued in the future.

A study carried out by Sally Sims and Peter Dent of the Department of Real Estate Management at Oxford Brookes University showed that visible powerline cables could reduce the number of potential buyers by up to 80 per cent, depending on the type of property concerned and the distance from the pylon or cable. It also extended the time it took to sell the house.[19]

Buyers were more bothered by pylons than by cables, especially if the pylon was to the front rather than the rear of the house.

Underground cables did not put them off so strongly, but this may be because some people in the study were unaware of their existence.

Up to 46 per cent of the buyers had problems with obtaining mortgages depending on the proximity and size of the power-lines near them. Valuers often underestimated the impact of powerlines on property, even though the lines could reduce the value by up to 38 per cent at 100 metres away, and the average reduction was about 11.5 per cent depending on property type, size and proximity to other features.

Reducing EMFs from powerlines

☺ If you want to buy a property near a powerline, or if you already live in one, you may want to think about reducing the electric field levels in the garden. The house itself will be protected because electric fields do not pass easily through building materials.

Planting trees will reduce electric field levels. Tree sap is conductive, so 'sappy' trees (some pines, cherry and so on) are better than non-sappy trees at reducing levels. Evergreen trees, which keep their leaves or needles throughout the year, are better than deciduous trees. Trees are slightly electrically conductive and help short out the electric field to the ground.

🗑 Practically, you can only avoid magnetic fields from power-lines – protecting yourself against them is very difficult. Lead sheets do not reduce fields, and steel sheets are not effective. A metal known as mu-metal does reduce the fields to a certain extent, but it is very expensive, and is hard to work with.

It may be possible – although unlikely – to get the powerline buried. Sometimes electricity companies will bury lines of 11 kV and below if local householders contribute most of the cost. In a few selected areas, energy network companies are gradually burying 230 volt overhead cables at their own expense as part of a general maintenance programme.

Keeping powerlines off your land

☺ In certain circumstances, you may be able to prevent a powerline from crossing your land. There are two forms of agreement that you may be asked to enter into by an electricity supply company, giving them the right to cross your land.

One is known as a permanent easement. This is an agreement whereby you give the electricity supply company the right, in perpetuity, to cross a part of your land in return for the amount of money specified in the agreement. When the land is sold by you to the next owner, the agreement is still valid. It must be attached to the property deeds, as it has legal implications for the value and use of the property. If you have bought land with such an agreement, you may be stuck with the powerline. We recommend you seek legal advice.

The other type of agreement is known as a wayleave. This is made between you, as landowner, and an electricity supply company, in which the company is allowed to install and maintain power supply lines and gain access for such purposes on a strip of your land. The width of this strip, known as a transmission corridor, depends on the voltage of the supply line and other factors and is specified in a notice issued by the company to you and in the wayleave agreement.

The wayleave may be for a specified length of time, often between 5 and 25 years, for a specific amount of money as annual rent. When you sell the land to another owner, the agreement has to be remade if that person wants to continue with it. By the same token, you should be told of any wayleave when you want to buy a property. Wayleaves should be attached to property deeds, or may be held by the landowner.

You may be able to prevent powerlines from being erected or buried on your land by refusing to enter into such agreements.

To get an existing powerline off your land, you need to give the electricity company notice to quit and ask that they remove the line. The company will then normally apply for a 'necessary wayleave' in which they plead that crossing this particular piece of land is the only reasonable way to provide electricity to other consumers. In most cases this will be granted to them, but if you can make the case for an alternative route, the company will have to justify why they can not use that. Cost can be a valid factor and you (or the seller of the property you want to buy) will probably have to pay part of the cost of moving the cables to the new route.

Removing cables beneath houses

Some cables (such as high-voltage power-supply cables and underground train cables) run in fairly deep trenches. These do not usually produce significant magnetic fields at ground level. Others are problematic, however.

🗑 Rarely, cables run shallowly underneath houses. This usually results in high magnetic fields. If this applies to you, you would need to seek legal advice as to whether the company can continue to supply electricity in this way, as the field levels would almost certainly be under international ICNIRP and UK guidelines (see page 21), although high from the point of view of research into health issues.

Houses built over shallowly buried cables were usually constructed without any consultation with the electricity company, who always try to avoid this. The situation may be illegal for safety reasons, and if you are the current owner, you may be required to have the cables rerouted, which can be very expensive.

We have come across two examples where house extensions were illegally built over existing underground cables and the problem was passed on to new owners. Such details should be checked for in the searches done when you are thinking of buying a property – ask your solicitor to obtain a plan of the underground electricity distribution cables in the area around your proposed house and check that supply cables to other properties all stay outside the boundary of your house. Usually, cables run close to the house boundary – especially under a common access driveway.

Reducing your exposure from powerlines and cables

DO

✔ Check the distance from the nearest overhead powerline. If your home is within the guidelines described in the box on page 43, measure the EMFs to check the field levels in your home and garden.

✔ If they are higher than the guidelines, see 'What you can do to reduce EMFs', above.

✔ If you have no front garden, or you are in a ground floor or basement flat, check the magnetic field levels in the rooms. Find areas of low EMFs for beds and chairs where you sit for extended periods of time.

✔ Ensure that people who may be vulnerable to EMFs sleep in levels of magnetic fields less than 0.1 microtesla and electric fields of 15 volts per metre or less.

✔ Make sure garden play areas and patios are in low EMFs.

✔ Plant trees to absorb electric fields if these are high.

✔ Check whether the price of a property you may be thinking of buying (or selling) reflects any discount due to the proximity of powerlines, pylons or cables. Also consider the likely effect when you come to buy or sell.

✔ If you have a powerline crossing your land,
check if there is a current easement or wayleave
agreement. Seek advice if there is not one, or a
wayleave has expired and you want the line
removed. You are likely to have to contribute to
the cost of moving a line.

DON'T

✘ We do not advise buying a house with cables
running directly overhead. These will usually give
high fields inside the house and may affect your
immune system's ability to keep you healthy.

✘ Do not go close to field crop spraying if there is
a high-voltage overhead line nearby. Recent
evidence shows that the toxic aerosols become
charged and are more likely to be absorbed by
your body.

Substations and transformers

Many people describe a substation as a 'transformer'. In this
book we define a substation as a collection of electrical equipment that includes at least one transformer and some
switchgear and protective devices such as fuses.

Transformers – so called because they transform voltage
from high to low, or vice versa – generally consist of two
coils of wire wound on two sides of a core that's made of
steel. One coil of wire is the input coil, through which the
electricity comes in; the second is the output coil, where it
goes out.

The 'transformation' of the incoming electricity can be dramatic. In the UK, the incoming voltage from the electricity supply system is generally 11,000 volts in residential areas, while as we've seen, the outgoing consumer voltage is usually 230 volts for a normal single-phase supply. Europe is now standardising the consumer voltage at 230 volts.

The main voltage and frequencies vary slightly around the world but we do not think this makes any significant difference to the issues raised here.

In towns and cities, you can often find substations every 150 metres. Substations that supply electricity primarily to a limited number of residential properties may look like brick sheds or walled-off yards, with a bright yellow and black 'Danger of Death' sign prominently displayed. Generally, they're not regarded as objects of beauty even by the electricity companies that own and maintain them. More importantly, they carry a risk of electrocution if someone gets in and touches the wrong thing by mistake, which is why they are closed off.

Larger ones – which can consist of several structures in a walled-off complex – may feed an industrial estate, a mixture of commercial and residential properties, or a large institution such as a hospital. Larger substations are associated with higher EMFs.

There are some enormous substations on the outskirts of towns – complicated structures bristling with electrical equipment and lots of transformers covering quite a large area of ground. It is not a good idea to live within 100 metres of one of these.

The higher voltage lines going to the substation from the grid may be overhead or underground cables. Those leaving the substation to supply an area are usually underground in large towns and cities, but may be a mixture of overhead and underground in more rural areas.

Our recommendations

Onsite substations
☺ Many schools have their own substation in the grounds. These are often near storerooms, and will present no health concerns. If your child's school has a substation next to a classroom, however, it may be a good idea to measure the magnetic fields, which will travel through the walls. Make sure that cupboards are placed between the wall and the classroom occupants so that no one is exposed to magnetic field levels above the 0.2 microtesla precautionary limit.

▥ Some business premises, offices, flats and houses (especially in urban areas) have substations in the basement of the building, or a substation may be attached to it. It is very important to find out if this is the case, as the floor above or next to the substation will usually be subject to very high magnetic fields. These are likely to affect the health of susceptible people, and can also cause computer display 'wobble' – which is against Health and Safety at Work regulations and can make operators feel ill. To affect a standard computer display, magnetic fields are likely to exceed 2 microtesla, or 10 times the level of our precautionary limit. Flat-screen TFT monitors avoid the 'wobble' problem, but still leave the operator exposed to higher than usual magnetic fields.

Local substations
You may want to investigate the area near your local substation to help find out how close the main cables are to the boundary of your land or house. The local electricity board can provide you with a plan of the cable layout. The company may

only supply these to a property's owner, so some negotiation may be necessary if you want to find out about a property you don't own. Cables may run under pavements, or the side of rural roads, and give surprisingly high fields when you take measurements directly above them.

☺ Often a substation, even next to a house plot, is separated from the house and/or garden by a passage or garage. We don't think that simply walking through high EMFs is likely to cause serious health problems, except for pregnant women (see below).

🗑 Pregnant women should avoid on-off exposure to EMFs in the first three months of pregnancy, as recent research (see Appendix), shows that sharp changes in magnetic field levels are associated with an increased risk of miscarriage.

Pole-mounted transformers

Transformers in rural areas often take the form of smallish, usually grey, boxes attached to a pole or poles of the (usually 11 kV) line that brings electricity to the area.

☺ The fields from these transformers fall off very rapidly and are usually negligible even 3 metres away. It's usually the fields from the overhead wires that are more of a concern, and we recommend that the 11 kV wires should pass no closer than about 20 metres of the house.

Problems with currents from substations

🗑 Substations are connected together, to ensure that, as far as possible, there is no disruption in consumer electricity supply. To attempt to provide a consistent voltage, the electricity company can connect substations in such a way that a high 'net' current is produced. This is current that comes from one substation and returns to another.

A net current doesn't have an opposite and equal balancing current in the cable running alongside it. This means it produces high magnetic fields that fall off slowly. This kind of interconnection is perfectly legal and an accepted practice within the UK electricity industry today, but it is problematic: it can create very high magnetic fields in houses. As electricity companies are not convinced this causes problems, there is little you can do about the problem through negotiating with them.

The only way to find out if your house is in the way of a net current is to measure magnetic fields at the house, preferably at a 'busy' time such as 8am or 6pm. If there is no net (or stray, see below) current problem, the magnetic fields should fall off very rapidly as you move away from where the cables are (usually under the pavement or roadway), typically falling to less than about 0.1 microtesla within a few metres.

If there is a net (or stray) current in the street, the magnetic field levels will only vary slowly as you move through the property, and not lower much with distance from the pavement or roadway. This can be anything from hardly changing at all, to falling by a factor of 2 or 3. High *electric* field levels near inside walls will be due to house wiring faults, not a net current (see Chapter 4).

🗑 'Stray' currents are caused by faults in the neighbourhood electricity system that cause electric currents to flow on metal gas and/or water pipes and give rise to higher than usual magnetic fields. When you are checking the magnetic field levels, if you find high fields that get stronger as you get closer to internal gas or water pipes, then stray currents are the likely cause.

Stray currents are surprisingly common. They can be stopped, although not always easily, and there is a cost involved.

The procedure usually involves inserting a short section of plastic pipe into the metal gas or water pipe close to where they appear from under the ground and come into the house, as shown in the figure below.

This is a job for the professional. Metal pipes inside the house still need to be earth bonded – or 'earthed' – to prevent electric shocks, as specified in the UK Wiring Regulations. The incoming pipe should be isolated as near the ground as possible, and any exposed pipe must be covered with insulating tape or sleeving, as under fault conditions it could give rise to a voltage shock hazard.

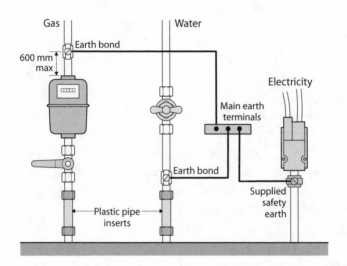

Reducing stray currents by isolating incoming metal pipes

Sometimes stray currents come into metal-framed buildings through the girders that extend into the ground. This needs professional help to deal with.

In some countries, stray currents are much more common than in the UK, as the electricity companies do not install a neutral ('return') conductor and use the earth to carry the return current. The problem is that if there are any metal pipes in the ground, the current often prefers to travel along them rather than through the earth.

Reducing EMFs from substations

☺ Most modern substation equipment for residential areas is enclosed in earthed metal boxes that do not give off electric fields. Any remaining electric fields from wiring are reduced dramatically by the brickwork, woodwork, railings and so on that are likely to surround the substation equipment.

Large substations that have exposed wires do emit electric fields, but these fall off rapidly with distance. Trees and bushes, especially evergreen or 'sappy' ones, will absorb much of the electric fields. These do not seem to affect the health of plants, so if trees or shrubs nearby are in poor condition, this is much more likely to be down to soil quality, rainfall levels and the like than electric fields.

🗑 Reducing magnetic fields is, as we have already seen, much more difficult. Magnetic fields penetrate all building materials and are unaffected by trees and bushes. The only things that effectively reduce magnetic fields are the internal design of the substation, such as the transformer, the cable layout and so on, and your distance from the substation. We always recommend that you check out the background magnetic field levels if you are thinking of buying, or renting, somewhere new to live. Net and stray currents (see above), for instance, can flow a long way from any given substation, so distance alone is not a good indicator of safety.

🗑 If you live in a bungalow, ground-floor flat or other single-story accommodation and there is a substation close to a bedroom, it is very important to measure magnetic field levels.

Until you have done so, put any beds in the room as far as possible from the substation wall, with the bedhead at the point furthest away. Remember that our guidance level for magnetic fields (which cannot effectively be reduced by screening) is below 0.2 microtesla maximum. Ideally, it should be no higher than 0.1 in bedrooms and less than 0.15 microtesla in play or sitting areas.

🗑 Do not build a patio, a child's play area or anything else where you or members of your family will want to spend a lot of time, next to a substation wall. Do not put a pram where a baby sleeps next to a substation enclosure.

☺ Thorny bushes such as roses planted in the garden next to a substation can keep people, especially children, away from areas of high magnetic field levels while they also help absorb electric fields. Ensure that any trees you plant to screen your house from electric fields emitted by substations or transformers are not used for leisure activities – so don't hang rope swings or hammocks from them, or build tree houses beneath or among them.

Reducing your exposure from substations and transformers

DO

✔ Measure the magnetic field levels close to your home. Remember the precautionary guideline levels of 0.1 microtesla in bedrooms and 0.15 elsewhere in the house. 0.2 microtesla is acceptable in the garden, as less time is usually spent there.
✔ Arrange the furniture in your house so that people sleep and sit in areas of low EMFs.

✔ Check where your nearest substation is. Get a plan of the underground cables between the substation and your home.

✔ Check your work environment for proximity to a substation and to the electrical intake/plant room.

✔ Check around any pole-mounted transformer, paying special attention to where the overhead wires are.

✔ Substations next to alleyways or cables running under passageways causing raised magnetic field levels are less of a problem because you are only exposed briefly to them. However, it is probably a good idea for pregnant women to avoid them.

✔ Measure your home for 'stray' and 'net' currents. If you have these, it could explain illnesses that don't go away. Take action to reduce any stray currents (see pages 56–7).

✔ Plant thorny bushes both to absorb electric fields if necessary and to prevent children playing in areas with high magnetic fields. Plan children's play areas and patios in areas of low EMFs.

✔ Check whether the price of a property you may be thinking of buying (or selling) reflects any discount due to the proximity of a substation. Also consider the likely effect when you come to buy or sell.

DON'T

✗ Avoid buying a house with a substation in the basement or in the garden.

✗ Avoid buying a house affected by a 'net' current.

> ✗ Do not place beds next to an outside wall with
>   a substation close by on the other side.
> ✗ Do not build a children's play area or a patio
>   next to a substation enclosure.

Mobile phone masts

Mobile phone masts (called 'base stations' by the network operators) are what enable mobile phones to work. They come in many shapes and sizes (see below), but all are equipped with the transmitting equipment that provides the signal that, in turn, keeps mobile phones 'talking' to each other.

According to the Mobile Operators' Association (MOA), in 2005 there were approximately 45,000 masts in the UK – a number that is set to rise to 50,000 by 2007, the deadline for the networks' requirement of 80 per cent overall coverage of 3G/UMTS. The masts carry signalling equipment for the different mobile phone networks and services and the TETRA system used by emergency services (primarily the police at the moment, though the other services are also being equipped). There are also some masts on railway property that are primarily used for rail network communications but can also be used by mobile phone companies.

Know your masts

The many faces of masts

Some masts are lattice structures with vertical antennas (which transmit a signal into the nearby area for phone users and cause most microwave irradiation), and dishes or drums (which send signals between masts and do not add significantly to the microwave exposure in their vicinity).

Other masts resemble tall, slim lampposts and are relatively unobtrusive. Yet others have been 'hidden' so they look like a part of a building, a burglar alarm, an attachment to a CCTV camera, a feature on a church tower or steeple, part of a petrol station sign, a tree, or any one of a multitude of imaginative ideas.

There is at least one company in the UK whose business is hiding mobile phone base stations so that they do not look like masts. Operators are fixing them to private houses on rainwater downpipes, or behind false burglar alarm boxes, in return for rents of thousands of pounds. You should be aware that any one of your neighbours may have found this offer hard to resist.

Why hide them? Not only are tall masts unsightly; the growing body of evidence about the risks of radiation from them has also understandably made many people reluctant to have them 'in their backyard'. More on that in a moment. First, let's look at how mast radiation behaves, depending on where the mast is sited.

How mast radiation behaves

The main microwave beam from an antenna radiates sideways, in some ways similar to a lighthouse beam. Most masts have three sets of antennas, each set covering 120 degrees out of the 360. Sometimes you will see what looks like just one cylinder on top of the pole. This is called a radome and it will almost certainly contain the three sets of compact antennas.

The main beam of radiation usually reaches ground level between 80 and 250 metres from the mast itself, depending on its height, how the antennas are tilted (both physically and electronically), whether the land is level or hilly, and whether there are buildings in the way. The upper floor of a building will be irradiated more by the beam than the lower floors, unless the building is higher than the antenna.

Some localised 'hotspots' of high radiation are detectable much nearer to the mast than the 80-metre distance suggested for the main beam. This is because antenna design is imperfect, and some energy is sent into 'sidelobes' of radiation as can be seen in the following diagram:

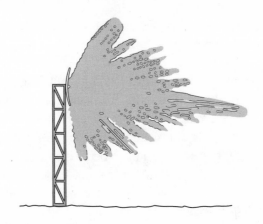

When masts are put on top of high buildings, and there are other high buildings nearby, the microwaves can bounce from wall to wall, exposing the people on all floors to unpredictable levels of radiation.

We saw earlier how mobile phone networks frequently hide masts to avoid community opposition, which often arises when planning permission is sought to erect a new mast or upgrade an existing one. Despite reassurances from the companies that the masts will not 'cook' nearby residents and are therefore completely safe, anecdotal evidence from people living near them, and a burgeoning body of research, are showing that the low levels of microwave radiation emitted by the masts affect a large and apparently increasing percentage of the population at levels well below those capable of heating tissue. Sometimes the research looks at distance from masts and sometimes the actual exposure levels are measured.

You are 3 times more likely to develop cancer if you live within 400 metres of a mobile phone mast in Naila, a town in Germany.[20] Living in field levels of 0.2 volts per metre from local masts – 300 times lower than the UK permitted level – causes the people of Murcia, in Spain, to suffer from depression, fatigue, concentration loss, appetite loss and heart and blood pressure problems.[21]

At the moment, planning permission in the UK is usually only needed for base stations over 15 metres high. As a result, the networks have started putting up masts at relatively low heights above the pavements of residential areas as 'street furniture', thus avoiding the need for planning permission and the associated public objections that go with the notification procedure.

How masts affect health

As we saw earlier, the organisation advising the government, the Health Protection Agency's Radiation Protection Division (HPA-RPD), states that microwaves are not considered dangerous if they do not have enough power to heat you. HPA-RPD has thus set a very high safe limit for microwaves known as the ICNIRP guideline. Some other European countries do not follow this guideline, and have now set far lower precautionary levels for mobile phone operators to work within – which they can easily do and the mobile phone handsets only need to receive a signal from the mast of less than one-billionth that of the ICNIRP exposure guideline level. Russia and China have also set low levels, though there is significant European pressure on them to increase their more precautionary guidelines to the ICNIRP level to help 'global free trade'.

Many very eminent scientists across the world believe that there are biological changes and adverse health effects on people, animals and plants at levels of microwaves millions of time lower than ICNIRP limit (see table below). We have added a column with volts per metre translated into a 'notional speed' in miles per hour based on a conversion of 30 mph as being equivalent to 0.6 V/m. This may enable you to better imagine the large range of views about what is safe and what is dangerous.

Public exposure guidelines for microwave radiation

National and Regional Guidelines 1800MHz	uW/m2	Equiv. V/m	Equiv. speed mph
NRPB prior to IEGMP (Stewart) Report	100 000 000	194	9479
ICNIRP (1998), WHO (UK 2004)	9 000 000	58	2847
Belgium (ex Wallonia)	1 115 000	21	1002
Italy (sum of frequencies)	100 000	6	300
Russia, PRChina	100 000	6	300
Switzerland, Lichtenstein, Luxembourg	95 000	6	292
Belgium Wallonia	24 000	3	147
Wien (sum GSM)	10 000	1.9	95
Italy (single frequency)	1 000	0.6	30
Salzburg 1998 (sum GSM)	1 000	0.6	30
EU-Parl, STOA GSM (2001)	100	0.2	9
Salzburg GSM/3G outside (2002)	10	0.06	3
Salzburg GSM/3G inside (2002)	1	0.02	1
Bürgerforum BRD waking (1999)	1	0.02	1
Bürgerforum BRD sleeping (1999)	0.01	0.002	0.1
Mobile phones can work at about	0.000 002	0.000 03	0.0015

Very little research has been, or is being, done in this country and internationally on the sort of pulsing microwave emissions that people are exposed to from mobile phone masts. However, there is already sufficient evidence to believe that they may affect health at least in a proportion of the population (see the box below), and until more evidence is available, we suggest that people take appropriate precautions. For more information on the research that is available, see the Appendix.

Reported health effects from mobile phone mast radiation include:

- Sleep disturbance
- Headaches
- Skin problems
- Nosebleeds
- An increase in the number and/or severity of epileptic fits
- Mood changes
- Behavioural disturbances
- Concentration problems and memory loss
- Heart and blood pressure changes
- Cancer
- Motor neurone disease.

Our recommendations

Equipment cabins
The radiating antennas on mobile phone masts are powered by electrical equipment housed in an equipment cabin.

Quite high levels of both mains electricity and microwave fields may be found close to them. The cabins may happen to be sited at spots where young people congregate, or where mothers linger with children in pushchairs, and may even be placed at a height that makes it a convenient perch. This is especially true of the cabins that feed lamppost-type masts. It is not a good idea to spend much time close to an equipment cabin.

Locating masts

You can find out where most masts are by looking on the government website www.sitefinder.radio.gov.uk. It is not entirely accurate, but it is the best we've got. The website is updated approximately every three months, so a mast that has only recently been integrated into the national network, or is only proposed, will not be on the site. The information on this website depends on the accuracy of the information given by the mobile phone operators to the people who enter it on to the database.

🗑 When locating masts in your area, remember that high-power masts sited at a relatively low level are usually worse than masts sited higher up when it comes to the amount of radiation that people living or working nearby are exposed to. Antennas attached to the walls of buildings can result in high field levels inside the building, on the other side of the wall. We have measured some office desks in London with over 3 volts per metre all around them from microcell base-station antennas mounted on the wall outside. Across the road, the pulsing microwave fields can also be very high depending on the power being beamed out by the antenna.

Operators are required to give their plans for masts for the coming year to every local planning authority each autumn. You have the right to ask to see this information at the local council offices, but you do not have the right to take a copy away with you – though some councils will provide one for a fee.

Local planning authorities do not co-ordinate planning consent applications among themselves. If you live on the boundary between two district councils, you may find that an application for a mobile phone mast is being considered by the council next to yours. If consent is given, the mast could later be made available to other companies to share the site, the mast or the equipment.

Masts and schools

There has been a lot of publicity in the press about mobile phone masts on schools. At least in part, this is because the *Stewart Report*[22] expressed uncertainty about whether mobile phone masts were 'safe' and suggested that as a precautionary measure, schools should not be in the main beam of a mast. The committee producing the report was headed by Sir William Stewart, ex-Chief Scientist of the UK and now the Chairman of the UK Health Protection Agency, and he has repeatedly stated the need for a precautionary approach being applied to mobile phone technologies.

> **The precautionary principle is now generally expected to be applied where scientific evidence is insufficient, inconclusive or uncertain and there are indications, through preliminary scientific evaluation, that provide reasonable grounds for concern that there may be some potentially harmful effects on the environment, human, animal or plant health. Where action is deemed necessary, measures should be: proportional to the chosen level of protection, consistent with similar measures already taken, based on an examination of the potential benefits and costs of action or lack of action and subject to review in the light of new scientific data.**

The Mobile Operators Association has devised 'Ten Commitments' to best siting practice. These suggest that schools which may be in the main beam of a mast should be consulted before the base station is erected. One in 10 schools have at least one mast nearby and Soho Parish School, in London, has 27. Most of these schools deny that they were consulted.

In 2001, one survey of young people under 15 at secondary schools reported that 87 per cent of them had their own mobile phones. This percentage is likely to have increased, rather than decreased, since then. Secondary school children are probably some of the heaviest users of mobile phones (despite the Department of Health guidelines that children under 16 should use mobile phones only in an emergency).

Many schools ban children from using their phones in school time. However, in the vicinity of any secondary school at the end of the day, there will be a dramatic upsurge in call traffic.

In fact, operators have had to erect masts near schools in order to meet the demand from the pupils using their mobiles. The networks are obliged by the terms of their licences to provide a signal for over 80 per cent of the population. Where there is a large amount of call traffic and inadequate signal capacity, more masts have to be erected to meet the demand. Often the best place to put a mast is on the school itself so that the masts do not radiate into school buildings. If the school refuses permission, the mast is often sited nearby, on privately or publicly owned land, from where it sends continuous radiation into the school buildings.

Although children at primary schools lag behind their secondary-school counterparts in mobile phone ownership, their number is growing. In January 2005, 25 per cent of

7 to 10-year-olds in the UK had their own mobile phone, despite the advice of the *Stewart Report* which recommends that children under eight should not use a mobile phone at all. This is an increase of 5 per cent since June 2004.

It is difficult to see how we can restrict the growth of mobile phone base stations near schools when so many children demand a signal for their phones.

Unfortunately, we are beginning to see the phenomenon of children calling or texting each other from one side of the playground to the other, or standing in a group not talking to each other, but busy calling or texting absent friends. It is almost as if they have forgotten how to hold an ordinary conversation with someone next to them.

Masts on railway land

Network Rail – which operates, renews and maintains the UK's rail infrastructure – and telecoms equipment company Marconi have joined forces in a project called Ultramast. Under this, the two bodies plan to put up a GSM (global system for mobile communications) mast every 5 to 8 kilo-metres along every railway line in the UK – resulting in about 2,500 masts.

🗑 Most of the masts will be at least 25 metres tall – the height of an eight-storey block of flats. Because of a legal loophole, they don't need planning permission, even in Areas of Outstanding Natural Beauty and in Conservation Areas.

Ultramast is intended, in part, to carry out improvements in safety communication that were recommended following the Paddington crash in October 1999, although a report published by the Health and Safety Executive estimates that the system used, the European Rail Traffic Management

System, will prevent no more than 16 fatalities in 40 years, at a cost of £267.5 million each. This seems an extremely expensive precautionary option compared with the lack of precaution regarding possible EMF hazards.

The railway communications are likely to be directional, following the line of the railway tracks. However, Ultramast are allowed to sublet space on their rail masts to any of the normal mobile phone operators. It is not clear whether this would require planning permission, but even if it did, local planning authorities are encouraged to allow mast-sharing, especially on existing structures. Unfortunately, for maintenance reasons among others, sites may be selected at existing stations – and this could be in the middle of a residential area or next to a school.

Masts and house prices

An increasing number of people report that their house has become unsellable because it is near a very prominent mast. So far, there has been no real research into this issue.

A couple called Philip and Nancy returned from a posting abroad to find a mast next to their bungalow in the UK. The mast was covered with new antennas – both for normal GSM mobile phones and for the Police TETRA communication system. Nancy's multiple sclerosis (MS) has become much worse and they have both developed electrical sensitivity. MS is a central nervous system disease where the electrical nerve signals do not pass properly around the body. Although it has not been directly associated with EMF exposure, there are quite a lot of anecdotal reports from MS sufferers that mobile phones and masts seem to adversely affect their well-being. Philip and Nancy are convinced that Nancy's condition is affected by the radiation from the mast next to their home.

Although they are desperate to sell and move away, Philip and Nancy have been told that the presence of the mast has at least halved the value of their home. Even with a much reduced asking price, Philip tells us that many people who come to view the house, arrive, see the mast, and immediately drive away.

As people are becoming more aware of reported health problems, soon it may not be just the visibility of the mast, but also the probable microwave exposure levels inside the house and garden, that could affect the market value of a property.

Reducing your exposure from mobile phone masts

DO

✔ Check whether there is a base station near you. They are not always visible. Try www.sitefinder.radio.gov.uk

✔ Remember that phones = masts. More phone use by you and your friends will *always* mean more masts and higher microwave levels in your environment.

✔ Measure the microwave fields with a suitable monitor – the Powerwatch Acousti-meter or the Electrosmog Detector (see Appendix). Ideally, the microwave levels should be below 0.05 volts per metre (V/m).

✔ Install screening measures if the microwave field levels are higher than 0.1 V/m, especially if you feel that you or members of your family are suffering the effects of microwave radiation sickness.

✔ Install screening measures if the microwave field levels are higher than 0.1 V/m, if you are considering selling a house near a mast.

✔ If your child is not performing as well at school as you were expecting, you may want to check whether there are high microwave levels from an external (or internal – see Chapter 7) source, affecting their ability to concentrate, learn or remember, or affecting their behaviour.

✔ Check that neither you, nor vulnerable people you know (including children), spend time near an equipment cabin supplying power to a mobile phone mast.

DON'T

✘ Don't buy a house just because there is no base station nearby. The mobile phone companies have got to provide good coverage for most of the population. If there is no mast at the moment, they may well need to put one up in order to meet the need of phone users.

Other outdoor EMF sources

TV and radio masts

So far, it has been generally accepted that there is little increased risk to human health from living near TV and radio masts. There have, however, been a couple of studies in the UK and Australia that have found an increased incidence of cancer around some sites near these masts. Some have queried whether these signals, when added to the pulsing microwaves from new mobile phone base stations, may be responsible for some cancer clusters. We know that the interaction between different forms of environmental pollutants is difficult to establish, as it is ignored by many of the authorities that make health and safety evaluations.

Ross Adey, the distinguished professor of neurology who made fundamental contributions to the emerging science of the biological effects of EMFs, complained that public pressure and funding bodies wanted rapid, simplistic answers to very complex problems.

Only limited short-term research programmes are being funded to answer specific questions about specific health risks. More complex or bigger problems are just not being explored – and many of the possible factors are not being investigated by anyone.

Radar equipment

Around the coasts of Britain, especially near major ports and Ministry of Defence establishments, radar can be a significant source of microwaves for a few nearby residents. Radar equipment is directional, so people living inland will not be as exposed as those along the coast.

People living near commercial and military airports and other MoD properties inland will also be exposed to microwaves from radar. The radio signal for radar is generally sent out in pulses, which can be detected by microwave monitors as a regular beat.

🗑 Studies of communities exposed to high radiofrequency from nearby radar stations in Latvia and Azerbaijan, compared with relatively low microwave fields in the neighbouring communities, found a number of negative effects on health, including reduced fertility and birth defects.

A three-year-old girl in St Andrews, Scotland, was diagnosed with and died of a neuroblastoma, a rare cancer which particularly affects young children. She lived near a TETRA mast (the police emergency services network) and radar from RAF Leuchars. Her mother says there seem to be more children with neuroblastoma in the area, than would normally be expected.

We were asked to survey the emissions from some mobile phone base stations round a rugby pitch in St Ives in Cornwall, because of general health concerns from nearby residents who were wanting to have the masts removed. However, we found that the dominant signal in the area surveyed was the coastguard radar from about half a mile away, which had been sweeping the area for the previous 30 years.

It is unclear whether combinations of high-frequency radiation, such as radar and other radiofrequency and microwave signals, may result in more health effects in the general population than either may independently.

You can reduce your exposure from radar emissions such as those from airport, seaport and coastguard services using a combination of special paint on the walls and screening material at the windows of your home (see EMFields in the Resources section). Military radar is sometimes a broader spectrum of pulsed radiation and more difficult to screen completely, though some reduction will be achieved using this technique.

Electrified railway lines

Many of the railway lines in Britain have been electrified, the power reaching the engines by means of overhead lines, or a third rail running parallel to the rails the train runs on. (For effects on drivers and passengers, see Chapters 5 and 6.)

Third rail power

An electrified railway line powered by a third rail will not normally create high EMFs in homes that are over about 10 metres away from the nearest rails. Houses built right next to the lines will be likely to have high transient fields when trains are passing nearby.

🗑 As railway systems are by their nature interconnected by the rails, they can be prone to 'net or stray error currents' where there are many lines within a few miles of each other, such as around Greater London. We discussed similar stray current problems arising in our normal electricity supply distribution, above. Some rail companies use direct current (DC) electricity to power their trains on their three-rail systems. This can cause a high magnetic field disturbance when trains draw power (that is, when the motors are actively pulling).

In one case we investigated in Petts Wood, Kent, the colours on TVs in houses about 30 metres from a railway line went haywire each time a fast train passed by – a clear indication of a severe magnetic field disturbance which might have long-term health consequences for nearby residents. This particular problem was due to the rail layout in the area and the location of the main electricity substation for the local railway lines. This created large DC net currents that caused the television tube colours to go badly wrong. A flat-screen (e.g. TFT, LCD or plasma) display avoids this problem, but the people would still be exposed to the transient fields – with unknown long-term health consequences.

Overhead powerlines on railways

Railway lines with overhead power are going to produce high fields near the lines themselves – both electric fields from the 25,000 volts on the overhead wires, and magnetic fields from the current being drawn by trains. As the metal rails and the overhead wires are separated by several metres, the magnetic fields travel a much greater distance than for three-rail systems where the rails are close together and the magnetic fields cancel out much better. All EMFs decrease with distance and have generally fallen off to background levels at a distance of between 30 and 50 metres, depending on the particular railway.

🗑 Homes closer than 30 metres to the overhead power cables feeding a railway may be subject to quite high levels of EMFs. We would advise measuring the fields if you are living, or planning to live, in such a location.

The effects of cuttings and embankments

☺ If the railway line is in a cutting, EMFs from a third rail are almost certain to be lower than if they were level with houses, as earth absorbs some of the electric fields. Overhead lines could be a problem if the house is close to them.

If the railway is on an embankment, fields from a third rail or an overhead line will only be reduced by the distance to the edge of the property boundary. The distance needed for EMFs to reduce is measured in a straight line between the overhead power cables and the property and its garden.

Living near a station

If a house is near enough to a station for passing trains to be slowing down or be in the process of speeding up, there are usually transient EMFs as the trains take power. When the train starts moving it draws the highest currents in order to accelerate. There has been some published scientific evidence that transient field levels (see also above) may be more problematic than continuous low levels, though it is an aspect of EMF exposure which has received little study and far more research needs to be done on these.

Security systems controlling access to buildings

People with electrical sensitivity can react very badly to the fields from the sensor systems and mechanisms controlling the barriers. They may not be able to live in, or visit, anyone living in properties where access is restricted in this way.

Because of concerns about transient exposures (see above), there may also be health effects experienced by people passing through these on a regular basis.

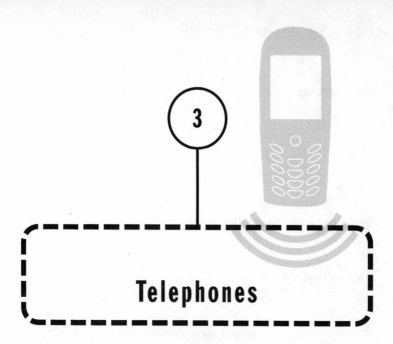

Telephones

Telephones are so useful that most of us can't imagine our lives without them. Invented over a century ago, the early land-line phone has gone through many changes and we now also have 'walkabout' phones – and many models of mobile phone. And it is these that have the biggest impact on your health, as we'll see in a moment.

Effects on health

As far as we know, the standard wired phone presents no concerns regarding EMFs for the vast majority of people.

There is mixed, but not unanimous, scientific concern about the health effects experienced by many people who use both cordless phones and mobile phones. (For information about mobile phone masts, see Chapter 2.)

The following effects on health have been found as a result of research into radiofrequency (microwave) radiation from cordless and mobile phones. The Appendix gives detailed information and references for research on microwaves.

Brain tumours – the longer you use a cordless or mobile phone, the greater the risk of a tumour developing.

Breast cancer – breast tissue in females *and* males very easily absorbs microwave radiation, increasing the risk of breast cancer.

Dementia – microwave radiation can kill off brain cells. As these never regrow, this can impair brain function.

DNA damage – microwaves can damage cells in ways that can pass on the damage to the next generation of cells.

Concentration problems and memory loss – microwaves affect the ability of the brain to process and remember information. This is especially important in children as their brains are still growing. In the short term, microwaves can stimulate the brain and improve some mental tasks but, in the long term, damage almost certainly occurs.

Behaviour and mood changes – chemical changes within the brain caused by mobile phone use may be responsible for aggressive behaviour and mood swings.

Fertility problems – the use of mobile phones has been linked to low and poor sperm count. The testes are highly absorbent of microwaves and a phone clipped to the trouser belt can result in considerable testicle exposure as the phone works on full-power at times when on standby and also when answering incoming calls.

Other possible problems – There is some evidence that microwaves can cause uveal melanoma (the most common form of eye cancer) and, at higher exposures, cataracts. If a mobile phone is clipped to a belt around your waist, microwave energy will be absorbed by your kidneys and/or your liver.

Our safety ratings

In the descriptions of specific types of appliance that follow, we use the symbols ☺ and 🗑 , in combinations of five, to show our assessment of its safety, and hence the level of care you need to take when using it.

For example, five 'smileys' – ☺☺☺☺☺ – show that that type of appliance is by far the best, whereas five 'bins' – 🗑 🗑 🗑 🗑 🗑 – mean that that appliance emits levels of EMFs so high that we recommend you don't use it.

You'll note that most of the appliances listed show a mix of smileys and bins. This indicates that they expose you to significant levels of EMFs when you're close to them – but if you keep a sensible distance away from them, they're probably fine to have around.

In other places where we discuss EMF exposure when, for example, you are travelling, we use a single ☺ or 🗑 to indicate whether there is likely to be a problem. Where *extra* care is recommended, we have used 🗑 🗑

Wired telephones (landlines)

Our recommendations

☺ ☺ ☺ ☺ ☺

The **landline telephone**, with a wire plugged into a suitable wall socket, is not a problem for most users. Note, however, that some people with extreme electrical hypersensitivity (EHS) can have problems using even this type of phone.

Cordless telephones

Our recommendations

🗑 🗑 ☺ ☺ ☺

With a 'walkabout' cordless phone, microwaves come from two places. With an **analogue cordless phone**, the base units only emit radiation while a call is actually being made. The handset gives off microwave radiation when in use, so calls should be kept short. The analogue system uses technology with a signal that does not pulse and, as most independent scientists believe that it is the pulsing that seems to cause most health problems, an analogue phone is likely to be safer. However, there is some evidence of brain tumours being more common among analogue phone users than among people who rely on landline phones, so it cannot be given an absolute all-clear.

🗑 🗑 🗑 ☺ ☺

Older digital phone handsets behave in a similar way to a mobile phone when you are making a call: the handset radiation pulses at a low but constant level. Health research has shown brain tumours to be associated with even minimal use.

Newer digital phones **(Digital Enhanced Cordless Telephone, or DECT)** are worse than older models. The base unit where the signal comes into the house sits and pulses out microwave radiation 24 hours a day, whether you are using the phone or not. The handsets also emit pulsing microwave radiation while you are using them, so if you use a phone standing near to the base unit you will get a double dose – one lot from the phone, and the other from the base unit. If you really cannot do without a cordless phone, get an analogue one, but not a new digital one.

Using landline and cordless phones

DO

✔ Use a traditional wired telephone for most calls
✔ Use an analogue cordless phone as a 'remote ringer', but go to a landline phone for the main conversation
✔ Keep your 'portable' phone calls short.

DON'T

✗ Don't have a DECT cordless phone in the house.

Mobile phones

Mobile phones are in use everywhere these days. Bear in mind that all mobile communications require base stations to support them and the more you use a mobile phone, the more base stations are needed. We look at what the science says about possible health effects in the Appendix. The two case studies below show dramatic personal accounts of what has happened to people who frequently used mobile phones.

One man used one, and sometimes two, mobile phones at once in his work as an installation technician for British Telecom. He was in his thirties, married with young children. After eight years of using mobile phones in his work, he was retired on health grounds: his memory was so affected he was unable to do his job.

In East London in the late 1990s, two young men bought mobile phones and were delighted at the free weekend talk-time offer that they had both signed up to. They used their mobiles between three to five hours per week for about a year and a half. They were then both diagnosed with Hodgkin's lymphoma, a cancer of the lymph nodes in the neck, on the side where they held their phone.

Our recommendations

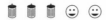

Mobile phones used in **emergencies only** can save lives and are an excellent way of providing key information to emergency services. Phones used in this way are unlikely to harm the user.

Mobile phones used for **texting only**, and held carefully (see 'Tips for safe use of mobile phones', below) are less hazardous to the user. Texting exposes you to lower levels of microwaves, but only because sending and receiving text messages does not take much time. Remember, however, that during that time you are still exposed to high EMF levels.

Mobile phones used **frequently or for long periods of time** are a definite hazard. Mobiles emit microwave radiation when they are in use, even when they are on standby. Microwaves penetrate the head, and the younger you are, the further into the brain they go, as the skull is thinner and brain smaller. Do not use a mobile phone for non-essential calls. Remember that the more calls you make, the more base stations are needed, especially in residential areas. As we saw in Chapter 2, base stations can cause significant ill-health symptoms in people living near them.

Tips for safe use of mobile phones

If you want to continue to use your mobile phone, the following tips will help you reduce your exposure to the damaging effects of microwave radiation.

☺ Your phone transmits at maximum power when you switch it on and off, when you dial out, when it connects or discon- nects, and when it is ringing. **Hold the phone away from your body** when you dial out and wait until the person answers before you put the phone to your ear. Hold your phone away from you when you finish the call. When you are texting, hold the phone away from your body to send or receive a message.

☺ Using a **hands-free kit** reduces the exposure to your head. It is important that it is the sort with air tubes, as the sort with wires to a headset can carry the microwaves to the brain as well. Be very careful where you hold the phone if you use a hands-free kit, as the phone will still be blasting out radiation wherever it is.

☺ **Keep your calls short**. This is good advice and comes from the UK Department of Health and an increasing number of governments across the world. Remember that you can talk to your friends as long as you like on an ordinary landline phone

– and with today's special tariffs and charge schemes, you won't be spending a fortune if you do so.

☺ Use a **pay-as-you-go tariff**. Although this works out as quite expensive per call, this will help you monitor the time you are on the phone and keep calls as short as possible. Different phone companies offer a huge variety of tariffs to get you hooked into using your mobile phone. ('Getting hooked' is an interesting phrase in this context because some research[23] has found that mobile phone radiation encourages the brain to release endorphins, the 'feelgood' chemical produced naturally – especially during strenuous exercise – in the pituitary gland.)

Ignore the temptation to subscribe to a service offering lots of cheap calls. Remember, the phone companies are making high profits which are coming from you, the user. Once you have committed to a monthly fee it is very tempting to make as many calls as they allow.

☺ Check the number of bars on your mobile phone – this shows how strong the signal is in the area you're in. If there is only one, you will get a poor signal and the call is likely to drop. Maximum bars gives you the best signal. When your phone is in a good signal strength area, it does not need to work so hard to keep your call going and it transmits using hundreds of times *less* microwave radiation. Using your phone only with maximum bars will reduce your exposure.

☺ Make a ring out of foam and use it as a 'spacer' to keep the mobile phone handset about a centimetre away from your ear. In this way you will greatly reduce the microwave power being absorbed by your head.

☺ Check where the nearest mast is likely to be when you make a call. If you know which direction it is in, hold the phone between you and the mast, so that microwaves do not go through your body during the call. If you are using your phone in a building, stand as near to the window as you can and hold the phone between yourself and the window. Ensure the phone can work using the lowest possible power.

☺ Mobile phones in standby mode 'talk' to the nearest mobile phone mast, possibly every few minutes, at maximum power. If you leave your phone in standby mode, it will be radiating the nearest part of you, or anyone else nearby, with high, even if brief, doses of microwave radiation. Unless you are sensitive to microwave radiation, you will be unaware of this – but it will be happening.

When your phone is on standby, put it in a bag or somewhere nearby, such as a table or desk. And whenever possible, **switch your phone off between calls**, so that you don't have to worry about standby radiation. (When you turn it on again, remember to hold it away from your body, and check in occasionally for messages.)

🗑 **Boys should not hold a phone on their lap** when sending or receiving a text message. As we've mentioned, testicles are particularly vulnerable to microwave radiation. Research has shown that microwave exposure can lead to fertility problems.

🗑 **Do not carry your phone on standby next to your body**, especially not clipped to your belt, or in a blouse or shirt pocket. If you do this you will radiate yourself with high doses of microwaves each time the phone 'talks' to a mast which, as we've seen, it does at full power on standby. The parts of the body most vulnerable to microwave damage are eyes, breasts and testicles, though all soft body parts are at risk.

🗑 **Do not carry your phone on standby in a bag hanging on a baby's pushchair**, next to the baby's head. They will be receiving a high dose of microwave radiation every time the phone logs on to the nearest mast.

🗑 **Do not stand close to someone making a call**. Their phone will radiate you as well.

🗑 **Never use a mobile phone (or carry it on standby) in a car or train**. Metal surfaces reflect microwave radiation and mobile phone signals bounce around all over the place often being absorbed by fellow passengers.

🗑 **It is illegal to use a hand-held mobile phone when driving.** A government project that looked into the potential hazards of driving while using a mobile phone found that it interfered with concentration as much as being over the drink-drive limit! This was true even of phones with a hands-free kit. Using a phone quadruples the risk of an accident happening in the next 10 minutes.

Although it is perfectly legal for a passenger to use a mobile phone, as we saw above, the microwave radiation will reflect off the metal body of the car and subject everyone in it to quite high levels of microwaves. If you want to make an emergency call, stop at the first convenient place and get out of the car to use the phone.

🗑 **Do not buy a mobile phone for your child or children.**
Children, because of their smaller head size and thinner skulls, are more likely to be damaged by the radiation from a mobile phone. Because of their age, they will be using mobiles for far longer than today's adults. Experiments on rats suggest that microwave exposure at a young age is associated with early-onset dementia.[24]

Parents often buy mobile phones for their children because they feel that they will be safe from paedophiles. However, a number of high-profile cases have shown that children who have had phones when abducted, and sometimes, tragically, murdered, have been unable to use them.

In a third of street robberies, a mobile phone is the only item stolen. According to the BBC in July 2005, 'Young people are especially at risk. When you are talking on your phone in a public place, you should treat it as if you are holding a £100 note to your ear, because some criminals will go to extreme lengths just to steal your phone.'[25] It is difficult to believe that possessing a mobile phone will really make children safer.

🗑 If you have **electrical hypersensitivity** (EHS), using a mobile phone is likely to make your symptoms worse, even when you stop using the phone. Our investigations into people's experiences show that you may become sensitised to other forms of electromagnetic radiation, or even chemicals and substances which provoke allergic reactions, though the mechanisms are poorly understood.

Some people with EHS cannot use even a landline phone without experiencing unpleasant side effects. As far as we know there are no UK manufacturers of telephones that can be used by this extremely sensitive section of the population. For more information on EHS, see Chapter 8.

Using mobile phones

DO

✔ Hold the phone away from your body when switching it on and immediately after dialling until the person answers.

✔ Use a hands-free kit (the sort with air tubes).

✔ Keep your phone calls short.

✔ Use a pay-as-you-go tariff, which encourages you to keep calls short.

✔ Only use your mobile phone when you have maximum bars showing (signal strength).

✔ Make a foam spacer for your phone.

✔ Hold the phone away from your body when you switch it off.

✔ When sending or receiving a text message, hold the phone away from your body.

✔ Always hold the phone between yourself and the signal source – such as between you and the nearest window.

✔ Switch your phone off between calls, if possible. Remember to check in for messages.

✔ Put your phone on standby in a bag, or somewhere close to you, but not next to your body.

✔ Switch your mobile phone off when travelling.

DON'T

✘ Don't hold a phone on your lap when sending or receiving a text message.

✘ Don't carry your phone on standby next to your body.

✘ Don't carry your phone on standby in a bag hanging on a baby's pushchair.

✗ Avoid standing close to someone who is making a call.

✗ Don't use a mobile phone in a car or train.

✗ Don't let a passenger use a phone while you are driving. Stop at the first convenient place, so they can get out of the car to use the phone.

✗ Don't buy a mobile phone for your child or children. The microwave radiation may be irreversibly damaging their brain cells or changing their behaviour. Using their phones may also make them targets of abuse – even putting their lives in danger.

✗ If you suspect you may be sensitive to microwave radiation, don't use a mobile phone. It is likely to make your symptoms worse.

✗ Don't use a mobile phone to watch films, play games or listen to music.

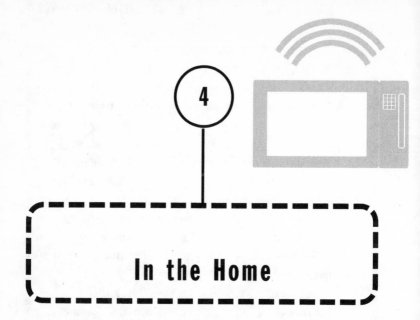

In the Home

We've now seen a number of reasons why you should minimise your EMF exposure. One of the most important places you can do this is in your own home. We spend much of our time at home if we include night time. Sleep is absolutely essential to us: our bodies use sleep to both manage and to carry out many of the essential repair processes needed to keep us healthy. There is good scientific evidence that the most important time to minimise our EMF exposure is while we are, or may be, sleeping.

With some care, it is often relatively easy to keep EMFs at a reasonable level in your home.

Kitchen appliances

Most kitchens contain a range of electrical and microwave appliances that produce EMFs. Healthy adults will remain relatively unaffected by levels in most kitchens. The people who are **most vulnerable** to EMFs are pregnant women, children, convalescents, men with a family history of testicular or prostate cancer, women with a history of breast cancer, and people with poor immune systems.

We believe that if you are likely to be pregnant, you should minimise the use of electrical appliances that sit on worktops, especially during the first two trimesters (see also Chapter 7). If you have a degree of electrical hypersensitivity (EHS), you are likely to react to all electrical appliances and should be close to them as little as possible (see also Chapter 8).

Our recommendations

Cookers

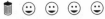

The standard electric cooker with an oven, grill and top plates gives off magnetic fields when it is operating. Vulnerable people should keep at least half a metre away from the rings/hob that are working, and a metre away from the ovens and grills other than when moving food in and out. Some halogen rings that we have measured seem to give off particularly high levels of magnetic fields, and are not recommended. If you have to use one, try to stand as far away from the heating rings as practical (at least half a metre) and avoid standing close other than when stirring the food.

The same rules apply to **fan-assisted ovens**, **double ovens**, **toaster ovens**, **grills,** mechanical **time switches** and so on, which also give off significant EMFs when working.

The fields from a **ceramic/glass-topped hob** can be lower than those from a traditional electric hob, but some **halogen** rings give off particularly high levels of magnetic fields and are not recommended. If you have to use one, try to stand at least a metre away and use at arm's length. They are best avoided if you are, or might be, in the early stages of pregnancy.

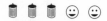

Magnetic induction hobs work on a different heating principle. The top of the cooker stays relatively cool and is mainly heated by contact with the hot pan. A few use 100 Hz, but most now use higher-frequency EMFs, usually between 18–23 kHz and 60-100 kHz, to induce currents into the pan.

There are two main types: those that only work with cast-iron and stainless steel pans, and higher-frequency ones that can also heat aluminium and copper pans. The EMFs they produce around the pan usually considerably exceed inter-national ICNIRP magnetic field guidance levels (up to 16 times above have been measured), but meet the basic ICNIRP restrictions for current induced in a person standing in the normal cooking position. Although induction hobs are very energy efficient and fast to use, we do not recommend that you use this type of cooker; they will induce significant levels of vibrating currents in you as you cook. There are also reports of people with EHS being made quite ill for some time after being in a room with a working induction hob. It is not known what such high oscillating EMF levels will do to the food being cooked, either.

The fields from a **cooker hood** motor can be high up to about half a metre away. Limit the time you spend in front of a cooker hood in the evening, as high fields near head height stop the production of melatonin (necessary for good health – see Chapter 1) for that night. If purchasing a new cooker hood, find out where the fan motor is and choose one with the motor as far away from your head as possible.

Microwave ovens are everywhere – and may constitute a real problem. There is evidence of biochemical changes to the structure of proteins and amino acids in foods cooked by microwaves and we believe it is important for all of us to avoid eating food cooked like this frequently. Most of us will inevitably eat such food when travelling and 'eating out', but we strongly advise against the regular use of a microwave oven in the home.

After some 20 years of research into their use, Soviet Russia banned the use of microwave ovens for heating food in 1976, as they decided that the dangers outweighed the main benefit, speed. They were allowed again from 1987 when, under Perestroika, Gorbachev allowed business pressure to change restrictive Russian regulations that did not fit in with free-trade practice in the West.

As well as changes to amino acids and proteins in food, it has been suggested that microwave cooking changes blood chemistry in the people eating the food in ways that ordinary cooking doesn't. The long-term health effects of these changes, if any, are unknown.

Increasingly research is showing that the packaging of processed foods for microwaving can release harmful toxins into the food. If you wish to use a microwave for cooking, we recommend that you turn the food onto standard crockery before cooking.

Microwave radiation **leaks from the seal around the door and through the glass** of microwave ovens. High (over one microtesla) powerfrequency magnetic fields extend for about a metre. Children should *not* be allowed to watch the food cooking, however fascinating the visible changes may appear. Microwave ovens have a sterilising effect, and those people who are having microwaved food because of being **treated for cancer** should stay out of the kitchen altogether.

If you choose to use a microwave oven, **heat food and drinks thoroughly** (which will help kill bacteria), and then leave to stand for two to three minutes before consuming. This is to allow re-absorption of free radicals – highly reactive chemicals which have a degenerative and sometimes carcinogenic effect in the body – and stabilisation of various compounds created in the microwave heating process.

Microwaving baby milk may be problematic. Dr Lita Lee reported in the 9 December 1989 issue of *The Lancet* that heating formula in this way converted some of the amino acids in it into synthetic forms that are not biologically active. One was converted to a toxic form. Lee said, 'It's bad enough that many babies are not nursed, but now they are given fake milk (baby formula) made even more toxic via microwaving.'

We do not believe that microwave cooking should be used regularly, especially for warming food for **babies** and infants who are so much more vulnerable. **Baby bottles** should *not* be heated to body temperature in a microwave oven and immediately given to babies. We do not recommend a microwave oven for the cooking or heating up of any baby or infant foods.

☺ ☺ ☺ ☺ ☺
Slow cookers usually use very low-power and do not pose a significant EMF hazard.

☺ ☺ ☺ ☺ ☺
Gas cookers do not use electricity and do not pose an EMF hazard. The sparks used to light the gas hobs do produce short bursts of high-voltage electricity, but these are also an insignificant hazard. Some people with multiple chemical sensitivity (MCS) have to avoid the fumes from gas burners.

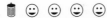

Electric steamers give off some EMFs (although not high levels) at worktop height. They are, however, a very good way of cooking food, retaining most of the vitamin and mineral contents.

A **deep-fat fryer** will give off high EMFs as the oil is heated. Regularly reheated oil is likely to contain carcinogenic compounds generated at the high temperatures, which will then attach themselves to the fried food. We recommend avoiding deep-fat frying for this reason, although from the EMF point of view, deep-fat fryers would probably only get a four-bin mark.

Other electrical appliances

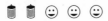

Small electrical gadgets such as electric kettles, coffee makers, food mixers, toasters, toasted-sandwich makers, bread makers and the like all give off EMFs at worktop height. If you are a child, elderly, pregnant or otherwise vulnerable, you should keep out of the kitchen as far as possible when these appliances are working. **If you are in the early stages of pregnancy, be cautious of using devices with electric motors (such as mixers and juicers) close to your body.**

Washing machines, dishwashers, tumble dryers, fridges and freezers all give off high EMFs next to the motor. If you are unsure where this is in the appliance, keep at least half a metre away from the equipment while it is working. As fridges and freezers are on all the time, it may be an idea to find out where the motor is (usually at the back next to the floor). It is important to bear this in mind if children, especially young ones who like to play on the floor, are often around this area. See also Chapter 7.

☺ ☺ ☺ ☺ ☺

A **freezer** has to work harder to maintain a low temperature if it is empty. Keep it reasonably full. A chest freezer is more energy-efficient than an upright freezer.

🗑 🗑 ☺ ☺ ☺

Ventilators and fans **can give off high fields at head height**. **Keep your distance at night**, because of the melatonin effect.

🗑 🗑 ☺ ☺ ☺

Floor **vacuum cleaners** give off high EMFs but are further away from your body than upright models. If you are pregnant, use upright models with care.

Reducing your exposure in the kitchen
DO

- ✔ Keep *at least* half a metre away from your electric oven when it is working.
- ✔ Minimise your use of worktop-height electrical appliances.
- ✔ If you are in a vulnerable group, prepare all the food for the meal and then minimise the time in the kitchen while the cooker is on.
- ✔ Check your microwave oven (if you have one) annually for microwave leakage from the seals. Remember that they also give off high levels of mains frequency EMFs within about a metre.
- ✔ Use an ordinary, halogen or ceramic hob in preference to magnetic induction hob plates.
- ✔ If you must fry food in deep fat, change the oil frequently in your fryer.

DON'T

✗ Do not use a microwave oven for heating baby milk or preparing other baby food.

✗ Do not use a microwave oven as your main cooking appliance.

✗ Do not let children stay in the kitchen when a microwave oven is on.

✗ Do not stand close to an electric oven or in front of a working cooker hood after dark.

✗ Do not allow children to play in front or beside a working oven, washing machine, dishwasher or fridge.

Lighting and wiring

Our recommendations

☺ ☺ ☺ ☺ ☺

Ordinary **incandescent bulbs** and non-halogen spotlights don't cause an EMF problem.

☺ ☺ ☺ ☺ ☺

Full-spectrum light bulbs are beneficial, especially as the majority of people do not get adequate exposure to daylight at work. They give out slightly higher levels of ultraviolet (UV) than standard light bulbs. Avoid using them after 10pm, when you should minimise all exposure to bright light because it will affect your body's melatonin production for that whole night. Red light, or weak yellow light, is acceptable.

🗑 🗑 🗑 ☺ ☺

Ordinary **fluorescent lights** give off high levels of magnetic fields up to half a metre from their ballast coils – these fields will go through the ceiling to any room above. The **flicker** and **hum** associated with these lights may be noticeable and trigger irritability, eyestrain and headaches. Some high-frequency, low-flicker, energy-efficient electronic-ballast fluorescent lights emit significant levels of very low frequency and/or radiofrequency fields, although modern high-quality fittings are usually quite good.

🗑 🗑 🗑 ☺ ☺

All '**energy-saving**' bulbs are high frequency fluorescents and can give off significant EMFs. Some also give off low-frequency radio waves. Make sure you use them in places that are not too close to people's bodies.

🗑 🗑 🗑 ☺ ☺

Halogen lights usually generate a lot of heat and need good ventilation if they are not to be a fire hazard. Most are low-voltage and so require far more current than mains-voltage lamps, generating higher magnetic fields. These are made worse by the 'suspended open-wire' systems they may be designed to hang down from, as the wires are quite far apart and run not far above an adult's head. Often these are not earthed, so they also give off quite high electric fields. To minimise electric fields, it is important that one side of the low-voltage supply coming out of the transformer is earthed.

Many low-voltage halogen light fittings have their own inbuilt transformer. Unfortunately, this is usually very poorly constructed and gives off very high levels of powerfrequency magnetic fields close to them. If set into the ceiling, with the light projecting downwards, there is not usually an EMF problem in the room being lit; but if there is a room directly above, then areas of high magnetic fields (from the inbuilt transformers) are produced in that room up to about 50 cm from the floor. If this is a child's room they are likely to be highly exposed when playing on the floor, and possibly even when lying on their bed or cot. One high-quality torroidal transformer (which will produce low levels of external magnetic fields) feeding all the lights on each circuit will avoid this problem.

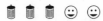

Halogen **desk lamps** usually have cheap transformers located in their base, which should be positioned at least 50 cm away from your body in order to minimise EMF exposure. Although they can produce attractive pools of light, it is important to position halogen fittings to ensure that you do not look at the bulbs directly, as they usually give off high levels of light in the blue part of the spectrum and quite high levels of ultraviolet radiation. Alternative types of desk light are recommended for places where you could be close to these fields.

> One man developed a case of central serous retinopathy when he looked to the side of a 20 watt *unfiltered* halogen lamp for about 15 minutes during a television interview. The back of his retina developed a blister and he lost vision over this area. Luckily, he recovered his full sight over a period of 18 months, but this kind of damage can result in permanent visual impairment.

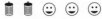

Anglepoise lamps and other metal-framed lamps can give off *very* high electric fields due to the practice of wiring lights with two-core flex. Always consider using three-core flex and connecting the earth wire to the metal frame.

Cheap (and older) **dimmer switches** and wiring give off radiofrequency noise, raising the overall levels of electromagnetic pollution. Most give off quite high fields up to a few inches from the light switch and wires. Instead of using a dimmer, consider having some lights with low wattage or coloured lamps to provide low-level lighting when required.

Incorrectly wired **two-way** hall/landing **switches** can give off high magnetic fields.

Most **standard lamps** and **table lamps** have only a two-core mains lead, which will give off high electric fields and should be kept well away from your body. Leads should be tidied safely away, running along skirting boards away from where you sit, wherever possible. This makes practical safety sense for children who spend a lot of time on the floor, and it also protects them from high electric fields from unearthed appliances, which are present even when the appliance switch is off. The wire of a table lamp should lead away from the person sitting next to it.

Reducing your exposure from lighting

DO

✔ Choose one high-quality torroidal transformer for each room where there are halogen lights.
✔ Keep halogen lamps away from the body.
✔ Have good ventilation in a room with halogen lights.
✔ Use full-spectrum bulbs if you spend a lot of the day in artificial light.

✔ Make sure that metal-framed lamps are earthed.

✔ Use screened cable for bedside lights and keep the lights as far away from your head as is practical.

✔ Switch off bedside lights at the wall if possible.

✔ Keep wires from standard and table lamps safely by the skirting board.

✔ Ensure wires leave lamps away from the feet of the person sitting near them, not under their chair.

DON'T

✗ Don't use fluorescent-tube desk lamps.

✗ Don't use halogen desk lamps with a built-in transformer.

✗ Don't use low-voltage halogen lights in a room directly below a child's bedroom.

✗ Don't look directly at a halogen bulb, even a low wattage one.

✗ Don't use energy-saving bulbs next to where people sit.

✗ Don't use cheap dimmer switches – these produce high-frequency EMFs on your wiring.

Bedroom electrics and appliances

It is vital to keep EMF levels in the bedroom as low as possible. As we've seen, it is at night that our immune system repairs the damage of the day and keeps us as healthy as possible. The fewer electrical and electronic devices in your bedroom, the safer you will be. Children's bedrooms are looked at in more detail in Chapter 7.

Our recommendations

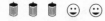

Bedside/bedhead lights give off high electric fields and the use of lights clipped to or built in to the bedhead is not recommended from an EMF viewpoint. As two-core cabling gives off electric fields even if the light is off at the switch, screened mains cable should be used, and the light switch should be away from the bed. Screened cable contains an earthed metal sheath to reduce electric field leakage. Reroute wires and use screened cable behind the bedhead if necessary, as the cables may increase electric and magnetic field exposure to the head. Keep the light as far away from your head at night as is practical. When you read late at night, use ordinary incandescent bulbs with as low a wattage as possible to avoid disruption to your **melatonin** levels.

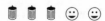

Beds with metal frames and bedsprings can become magnetised during manufacture and this has been reported as increasing the likelihood of cancer, multiple sclerosis and chronic fatigue syndrome, especially when higher than normal EMF levels are also present. Magnetised metal frames are also believed to cause increased restlessness and insomnia. Mattresses can be 'de-gaussed' (de-magnetised), although few companies do this.

☺ ☺ ☺ ☺ ☺

If you think your bed may be responsible for sleep problems, find a **non-metallic bed base and unsprung mattress**, preferably made of natural materials. Futons can fit the bill, but may take some getting used to as they can be much firmer than sprung mattresses.

☠ ☠ ☠ ☺ ☺

Waterbeds *can* give off high magnetic fields from the water heaters, though some do not. Ideally, the bed should be

warmed during the day and be unplugged before going to bed.
However, an unheated water bed can get quite chilly, so you
may need a thick mattress pad or quilt to stay warm. It is best
to avoid beds with a pumped heater unit attached to the foot.
Some anti-bedsore hospital beds are like this.

🗑 ☺ ☺ ☺ ☺

Electric underblankets used as directed – that is, *never* with a
person lying on them when they are on – are fine for
prewarming a bed before the person gets in. These blankets
are both an EMF and a fire hazard if turned on when
someone is resting on them.

🗑 🗑 🗑 🗑 ☺

Electric overblankets create a magnetic field that penetrates
thoughout the body, and most also produce an electric field.
They are designed to be left on all night, which results in high
and prolonged EMF exposure. Electric blankets can cause
cramp, and their use has been associated with miscarriages
and serious illness in children (see Chapter 7). Underblankets
and overblankets should *always* be switched off at the wall
before getting into bed. A tufted lamb's wool underblanket is a
good alternative – a natural, safe way of keeping warm.

Electric overblankets which are designed to be left on
overnight are usually run from a low-voltage transformer. Both
the transformer and blanket give off even higher magnetic
fields than underblankets. Do not use such a blanket if you
are concerned about EMF exposure.

🗑 🗑 🗑 🗑 ☺

Consider replacing electrical **heating pads**, used for chronic
pain relief problems, with hot-water bottles.

Where to place bedroom appliances

Always keep **electrical appliances** of any sort some distance (ideally **at least 1 metre**) away from the bedhead. If you have any closer than this, and it is impracticable to move it, switch it off at the wall, or unplug it, after use.

Wherever possible, do not run **electric wires** behind the bed, even along the skirting board. You could put them under the carpet and put earthed aluminium foil over the top. Use screened cable in the wall or metal conduit to reduce EMFs as near as possible to zero.

🗑 🗑 🗑 ☺ ☺

Televisions should always be **at least** 2 metres away from the pillow area. It is particularly important to earth TVs in bedrooms because of the high electric fields they usually give off. Battery-operated **remote controls** are quite safe. Switch TV sets off when not in use as they are drawing power even on standby – which aside from anything else is a waste of resources.

🗑 🗑 ☺ ☺ ☺

Clock radios should be kept at least 1 metre away from the nearest pillow, as they will be giving off high fields throughout the night. Older electro-mechanical clocks are worse than newer, electronic digital ones. If this is not possible, perhaps replacing it with a wind-up alarm may be a good idea.

🗑 🗑 ☺ ☺ ☺

As a result of the effects of climate change, our hotter summers can produce airless bedrooms that make it hard to sleep. So **electric fans** are increasingly used to keep the room cool. They contain an electric motor which gives off quite high magnetic fields. Some only have a two-wire lead and are not earthed, so they also give off high electric fields. Keep a fan at least 1 metre away from the bed.

🗑 🗑 ☺ ☺ ☺

Ceiling fans contain an electric motor which will give off quite high magnetic fields. You will not experience these in the room being cooled, but there will be a magnetic 'hotspot' in the room immediately above, extending outwards and upwards depending on the strength of the motor. If you live in a flat (or you have a ceiling fan in a downstairs room) with a fan directly beneath your children's bedroom, it is important not to let a child spend lots of time playing on the floor just above. Shops and restaurants sometimes have them, which may be worth bearing in mind if you have a flat above such premises.

🗑 🗑 🗑 🗑 🗑

The **charger unit** for your mobile phone gives off high levels of EMFs. Also, if the phone is left on standby it will broadcast microwave 'handshake' signals regularly during the night. Do not charge your mobile phone in your bedroom.

🗑 🗑 🗑 🗑 🗑

Do not keep your mobile phone on your bedside table. If you want to have the phone in your bedroom for emergency calls, keep it as far away from your bedhead as possible. Have an ordinary wired telephone in the bedroom and ask people to ring that number in emergencies at night. While the mobile phone is on standby, it will be radiating at full power quite frequently, depending on the strength of the signal available to it. (See Chapter 3 for more information about mobile phones.)

🗑 🗑 🗑 🗑 🗑

Light at night. There has been quite a lot of research which shows that exposure to light at night can seriously affect our immune system (see the Appendix). Most of the time we keep lights on at night to enable us to avoid tripping up in the dark or to help us keep a check on the welfare of the very young or the unwell.

🗑 ☺ ☺ ☺ ☺

Low power red or orange lights do not seem to significantly affect the pineal gland – which produces the melatonin that helps prevent cancer, boost our immune system, reduce depression and helps us sleep. So, if you feel you need a light at night to see by, we suggest that you replace the ordinary bulb with a low-power red or orange one.

Heaters

Our recommendations

🗑 🗑 🗑 🗑 ☺

Off-peak electric **storage heaters** may be used as your main form of heating. During the day they gradually radiate the heat that they absorbed during the night, cooling down as they do so, until they once again switch on in the small hours of the morning and the cycle restarts. During the daytime part of the cycle, the heaters give off heat, but no EMFs (unless you have a short after-noon 'top-up' period). At night, they give off quite high levels of EMFs during the charging-up period, which starts just after midnight. Allow at least a metre between the heater and a bed – and this includes where they are located on the other side of an internal wall! That also applies to dog and cat beds downstairs.

🗑 🗑 🗑 🗑 🗑

Avoid **electric floor heating** in bedroom areas. It may be used in other areas.

🗑 🗑 ☺ ☺ ☺

Fan heaters, oil-filled radiators and convection heaters all give off fields close by but if kept at least a metre away are usually fine. Fan heaters give off the highest fields because they have an unscreened motor to drive the fan.

Reducing your exposure in the bedroom

DO

- ✔ Keep beds as far away as practicable from electricity meters and immersion heater cupboards.
- ✔ Measure the EMFs if a bed is close to the meter cupboard, or if it contains wiring leading to other people's apartments.
- ✔ Keep beds at least a metre away from night storage heaters.
- ✔ Have a bed with as little metal in the frame and mattress as is comfortable.
- ✔ Use a hot-water bottle or fleece underblanket for extra warmth in bed, rather than electric blankets.
- ✔ Keep bedside lights as far away from your head as is practicable.
- ✔ Replace your bedside light's two-core cable with screened three-core cable.
- ✔ Keep TVs at least 2 metres away from your pillow.
- ✔ Keep clock radios at least 1 metre away from your pillow.
- ✔ Switch electrical appliances off at the wall.
- ✔ Keep your mobile phone as far away as is possible (if you have to have one at all in your bedroom).
- ✔ Replace light bulbs that are on at night with low-power red, orange or dark yellow ones.

DON'T

✘ Do not leave a waterbed heater on all night.

✘ Do not use electric heating pads for localised relief.

✘ Do not leave an electric underblanket on when you are in the bed.

✘ Do not use electric overblankets.

✘ Do not run electric wires behind the bed.

✘ Do not have a fan near the bed.

✘ Do not have your mobile phone charger in your bedroom.

✘ Avoid having lights on at night at all, if possible.

Audio/video equipment

Our recommendations

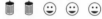

Televisions, as we've seen, give off high magnetic and electric fields up to 1.5 metres away. Regarding the level of EMFs, different models of television vary from make to make. Always sit *at least* 1.5 metres away from the front of the screen. Remember that magnetic fields travel through walls. EMFs from **digital TVs** are not much different in level from older analogue models, though some people with EHS say that they are more affected by them.

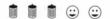

Televisions also generate **static electric fields**, which attract fine aerosol particles. Research from the University of Bristol (see Appendix) shows that these particles can have viruses, bacteria and carcinogens attached. These may be inhaled into the lungs or may stick to the skin. Children should sit at least 1.5 metres away from a TV screen to reduce this effect. The static charge persists for some time after the television has been switched off. The screen should be wiped with a *slightly* damp (or anti-static) cloth regularly when the television is off and the 'dust' carefully washed away.

Use the main switch on the set to switch off the television. Some types of remote control leave your TV on standby and it continues to consume up to a quarter of the energy it uses when fully switched on.

🗑 🗑 🗑 🗑 ☺

Plasma screens are sometimes used for large, flat-screen, wall-mounted displays. They can give off high levels of electric fields and people should watch them from a minimum of 2 metres away.

☺ ☺ ☺ ☺ ☺

These days, all **TV and video remote controls** work using very low-power infrared light, and pose no EMF problems.

🗑 ☺ ☺ ☺ ☺

There is only a subtle difference between **satellite dishes and receivers** and **digital TV receptors,** in the way the information is coded into the signal. TV reception signals are very low power indeed and are believed to have no biological effect. Digital TV receptors can give off high electric fields if the TV system or satellite decoder is not connected to the mains elec-tricity safety earth. Most TVs, video recorders and satellite systems are not earthed when you buy them, as they only have two-wire mains leads. Walls will give some protection from the electric fields; windows are less effective at screening them.

🗑 ☺ ☺ ☺ ☺

DVD and video players and recorders do not give off significant EMFs. Nor do Sky boxes or digital set-top boxes, though they should be earthed.

🗑 🗑 🗑 🗑 🗑

TV, video and HiFi **microwave transmitter boxes**, used to transmit pictures and sound from your main entertainment system to all other rooms in the house with a suitable receiver box, should be avoided where possible. They are another source of microwave exposure that you are deliberately bringing into your home environment. See if you can arrange your household's viewing without needing to do this.

🗑 ☺ ☺ ☺ ☺

Personal stereo players, MP3 players, iPods without Bluetooth or WiFi RF links are all fine.

🗑 🗑 🗑 🗑 🗑

You should avoid music players built into mobile phones. The standby signals irradiate you with microwaves while you are listening to music. Get a separate player and keep your mobile in your handbag or briefcase away from your body.

Computers and games consoles

Our recommendations

🗑 ☺ ☺ ☺ ☺

Computers (see also Chapter 5) have changed a great deal over the past few years. Some **computer display monitors** (VDUs) with cathode ray tube (CRT) type screens used to give off very high electric and magnetic fields from the screen and associated scanning coils. Early AppleMac colour screens emitted particularly high levels.

Newer, low-radiation displays complying with the Swedish guide-lines, adopted throughout Europe, give off far lower EMF fields over a range of frequencies (look for an MPRII, TCO92, TCO95 or TCO99 label on the back of the monitor). We still recommend that you sit *at least* 50 centimetres away from the front of the screen. Flat colour screens (known as TFT screens) are only a few inches thick and have very clear displays. They give off almost zero magnetic fields, though they can give off significant electric fields. Some users love these screens – some hate them and find they give more eye strain. All users should take at least one five-minute break away from their computer every hour.

All CRT VDUs give off higher fields at the back and sides. Always sit more than a metre from the rear of a VDU. Magnetic fields travel through walls, so watch the use of the next room. Smaller VDUs are not necessarily better, either, because the field's strength depends more on the internal design than on the screen size.

The casing and electronic components of a computer monitor contain fire-retardant chemicals that are released in use, mainly during the first few weeks when the warmth generated causes the chemicals to be released into the air. These can produce quite toxic side-effects and at worst could trigger EHS. If possible, switch it on in an unused room for about two weeks – otherwise make sure that your room is well ventilated.

Laptop computers give off very low EMFs. They can emit signifi-cant levels of electric fields from the back illumination and scanning processes. When run from the mains adapters they can give off very high electric fields next to the keyboard and display, of several hundred volts/metre. Charge laptop computers away from where you sit, and then run them off their internal recharged batteries, or earth the laptop.

The 2005 DELL Inspiron range of laptops came with a three-pin mains cable and an earthed adapter. These do not emit electric fields. Check for this kind of feature when you buy. Dell are to be congratulated on this change – to date, we know of no other manufacturer that does this. We suggest that you use the laptop PC on a table, rather than on your lap, as the underside gives off magnetic field pulses from the disk motor and a range of radiofrequencies. These are not good for male fertility and may help to trigger testicular cysts.

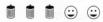

Computer games consoles such as the Xbox, Playstation, GameCube, Nintendo Revolution and so forth usually have a mains transformer which plugs into a power socket. The transformer gives off very high levels of magnetic fields, and should be unplugged when not in use. Often neither the TV nor the games controller is connected to mains 'earth', so the hand controllers can give off electric fields of several hundred volts per metre, but it does not seem easy to predict which ones do this. It is always worth measuring the electric and magnetic fields from such devices and adding an earth wire if the electric fields are high.

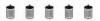

Computer wireless local area network (wLAN) broadband systems enable different members of a household to have broadband access for their portable laptop computers without needing to have a fixed source. Such 'wireless enabled homes' are filled with pulsing microwave radiation all of the time (even when the computer(s) is/are not in use), and we believe that you should avoid using these in your home at all costs. It is better to get a cable or ADSL modem/router and run network cables to the rooms where you wish computers to have internet access. This is not expensive and will avoid irradiating your home with pulsing microwaves.

A British dentist wrote to us of her experiences.

I linked the onset of my symptoms (heart arrhythmia, sleep disturbance, tightness in the chest, loss of energy) to our acquisition of a laptop with a wireless modem in the hallway. This 'base station' transmitted microwaves 24 hours per day for a radius of 40 metres. Other members of my family have been abnormally fatigued with disturbed sleep patterns, episodes of dizziness and vomiting. We disconnected the wireless base station, replacing it with a fixed line. Within three weeks our symptoms had disappeared.

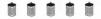

Most urban areas are well served by broadband through their telephone or cable networks. But many small rural telephone exchanges cannot yet handle the capacity needed for broadband (though coverage is spreading quickly now), and satellite access is expensive. So some companies offer **microwave broadband** facilities to villages, if there are enough subscribers to support the infrastructure. This will usually consist of a main receiver/transmitter attached to a house and then subsidiary transmitter/receivers at the other properties subscribing to the service. This will add to the overall microwave exposure for everyone who lives near the transmitters and receivers. There have also been many reports of customers dissatisfied with the connection quality – the systems use Bluetooth technology at the limits of its capability.

Hairdryers

Our recommendations

🗑 🗑 ☺ ☺ ☺

Handheld **hairdryers** use high currents to produce heat and to drive the motor. The motor gives off very high fields near the handle, dropping only a little at normal drying distances (6 to 18 inches). The fields are slightly higher when it is on a 'high heat' setting than when it is on a 'low heat' setting. Any metal pins and so on in the hair will distort the fields, increasing EMF exposure. The fact that a hairdryer is only turned on for a few minutes each drying session is not as important as the fact that the user is exposed to very high fields indeed while it is working.

We recommend that no hairdryers should be used after 7pm. High magnetic fields near the head in the evening are known to potentially interfere with the production of melatonin by the pineal gland for the rest of that night (see Appendix).

🗑 🗑 ☺ ☺ ☺

The heating units for **hair curlers** will give off significant EMF levels, although the curlers themselves are fine. Sit away from the heating unit while it is still working. When you have removed the curlers, it is a good idea to switch the heating unit off at the wall.

🗑 🗑 🗑 🗑 ☺

Hair curling tongs and flattening irons are self-contained heated units. The tongs will give off quite high fields, particularly electric fields. It is best to use them with care and not after 7pm in the evening, to prevent the fields interfering with melatonin production.

🗑 🗑 ☺ ☺ ☺

Hood hairdryers have a very high field, and the greater the heat setting, the higher the field. Sitting still under the hood regularly may have an adverse effect. Any metal curlers, or metal parts used in the curler construction, will increase EMF exposure.

☺ ☺ ☺ ☺ ☺

Wall-mounted hairdryers use a simple pipe to channel warm air to the head, so they're safe as far as EMFs are concerned.

Other leisure equipment in the home

Our recommendations

🗑 🗑 🗑 ☺ ☺

Electric **sewing machine** motors give off high magnetic fields, and some with two-core mains cables give off high electric fields. Statistically significant increases in the incidence of Alzheimer's disease have been detected in machinists using industrial sewing machines. There are some concerns about breast cancer. Be aware of where the motor is, and if you are elderly, pregnant or otherwise vulnerable, change to an old-fashioned treadle-driven machine if you plan to machine-sew for prolonged periods.

🗑 🗑 🗑 🗑 🗑

Most **sunbeds** give off high electric and magnetic fields as well as possibly dangerous levels of ultraviolet radiation. Many can give off five times as much UVA as would be expected from bright sunlight at the equator. If you use one, it will increase your risk of developing skin cancer, especially if you are fair-skinned.

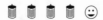

Sunlamps are all right as far as general EMFs go, but like sunbeds they give off ultraviolet light – a form of non-ionising radiation that we know causes skin cancers.

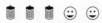

Exercise machines are generally not a problem. Remember that motors (such as those used to power treadmills) give off high magnetic fields close to. The exercise is probably more beneficial than the small level of potential risk.

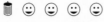

Some **Jacuzzis** have pumps and motors built into the base that result in high EMF exposure as you take a bath. We do not believe that short-term use in a hotel is a problem, but if you have a Jacuzzi in your house, we recommend that the pumps and motors are at least half a metre away from the bath.

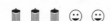

Vibrating **muscle toners** give off both electric and magnetic fields. This is probably all right if you are not electrically sensitive or pregnant, but normal exercise would be healthier.

TENS (transcutaneous electrical nerve stimulation) machines are used for chronic pain control and sometimes for muscle stimulation and toning. They work by passing short pulses of electrical energy frequently through parts of your body, usually through self-adhesive connector pads. They can be highly effective – the best ones have lots of adjustments and 'programme' settings. But it is inadvisable to use one if you are electrically sensitive.

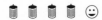

Two-wire (non-earthed) electrical equipment wiring is now in
common use Many electrical appliances come with two-wire
mains leads or adapters and are often described as being
double-insulated. This is done for a variety of reasons,
including protecting against electric shock. It is cheaper to
cover metal objects in plastic than it is to ensure good electrical earthing of exposed metal parts. The downside is that the
'workings' of all these appliances tend to radiate high electric
fields of often several hundreds of volts per metre nearby.

The worst offenders we have found are televisions, videos,
electronic organs, electric typewriters, some HiFi units,
portable computers when run off their mains adapter/charger
units, and battery chargers. Most of these can be cured of
giving off high electric fields by taking an 'earthing' wire from
their mains plug to an exposed screw or piece of metal on the
appliance.

In the case of electronic organs and HiFi units, the braid
screen of one of the audio cables is normally suitable for
making the earth connection to.

With televisions, the braid of the aerial lead usually makes a
suitable connection point. As televisions and video recorders
are usually connected together, it is not necessary to earth
both units.

In the case of portable computers, any metal connector shell
on the back of the computer will do.. It is often convenient to
use a 'crocodile' clip on the earth lead so that it is easy to
attach and detach when you need to move the computer. As
we've mentioned, the 2005 Dell Inspiron range of laptop PCs
are supplied with an earthed power supply.

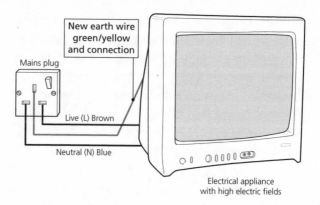

New earth wire green/yellow and connection

Mains plug

Live (L) Brown

Neutral (N) Blue

Electrical appliance with high electric fields

Reducing your exposure from audio/video and other leisure equipment

DO

✔ Keep at least a metre away from the front of a television set.

✔ Position a TV set so that the back and sides are away from where people sit or walk.

✔ Make sure your TV system or satellite decoder is connected to the mains electricity safety earth.

✔ Sit at least 50 cm from the front and more than 1 metre from the rear of a computer or games VDU.

✔ Ideally, take a five-minute break every hour when you are using a computer.

✔ Ideally, switch on a new computer monitor in an unused well-ventilated room for about two weeks before use.

✔ Earth your laptop, or charge the batteries and run it off them.

✔ Always unplug games console transformers when they are not in use.

✔ Think carefully before subscribing to a microwave broadband system for use with the internet.

✔ Try not to use hairdryers after 7pm.

✔ Use a wall-mounted airpipe hairdryer if possible.

✔ Use sunlamps minimally if at all.

DON'T

✗ Do not sit near the side or back of a television.

✗ Do not use a games console without first checking electric field exposure.

✗ Do not have a wireless network (wLAN) system in your home.

✗ Do not regularly use electric curling tongs to style your hair.

✗ Do not use an electric sewing machine for lengthy periods of time if you are in a vulnerable group.

✗ Do not use a sunbed.

Wiring in the home

We saw in Chapter 2 how substations, powerlines and other EMF sources in the outside environment can create high electric and, especially, high magnetic fields in the home. But over half the high EMFs in houses are due to wiring and electrical appliances. We have also found enormous magnetic fields resulting from currents flowing along 'earthed' pipework and metalwork.

Elevated fields within your home can aggravate, or may even cause, a number of chronic ill-health problems (such as depression, chronic fatigue and some cancers), but there is much you can do, or can have done, to prevent this.

It is, in fact, possible to wire buildings in ways that produce virtually zero electromagnetic fields. Often large modern commercial buildings have remarkably low fields from the wiring because all the wires are run inside metal pipes/boxes.

The electric field from normal three-core cable falls away fairly rapidly and, by careful routing, fields in critical areas (such as beds) can be kept fairly low even using normal cable. For the main wiring of a building, a system where the wires are contained in a screened cable or metal pipe reduces the external electric field from them to almost zero.

To minimise magnetic fields we recommend that 'ring final circuits', common in the UK, are not used and that they are converted into 'radial final circuits', such as those used in most of the rest of the world.

Field levels to aim for

To assess the present levels of electric and magnetic fields in your home, it will be necessary to obtain a suitable EMF meter (available for hire from EMFields, see Resources) or the services of an electrician who has an EMF meter and understands the concerns raised in this book. Such an electrician is not always easy to find, as in our experience, most have little knowledge about electric and magnetic fields.

A guide to typical 50Hz AC electric field levels

Electric field	Comments
< 10 V/m	With good design it would be easy to ensure AC electric field levels in the home below this level which we believe is generally OK for safety
5–25 V/m	The average in UK homes and therefore a level that can be regarded as 'normal' in the middle of rooms away from wiring and electrical appliances
>25 V/m	30–75 V/m can be regarded as the higher end of general background AC electric fields in homes. Near wiring and electrical appliances, electric field levels can reach several hundreds of volts per metre.

A guide to typical AC magnetic field levels (50Hz)

(international microtesla and USA milligauss units)

T	mG	Comments
0.05	0.5	The average in UK homes and therefore a level that can be regarded as 'normal'
0.20	2.0	The high end of what could be regarded as the normal range of fields in homes not near power-lines
0.40	4.0	The magnetic field level (when present as a 24-hour average) associated with a doubling in incidence of childhood leukaemia, even though a causal link is not proven. This level of residential magnetic fields may be too high for the long-term health of susceptible people.

In most homes, electric field levels less than 10 V/m from *internal sources* should be reasonably achievable in most of the rooms and should be fine for everybody who is not electrically hypersensitive (EHS). Some EHS people require electric fields to be almost zero. The electric field can be hard to reduce because of the way many houses have been wired.

Automatic 'demand switches' (see below) can be useful as a remedial measure. Remember, electric AC fields inside houses are usually the result of internal wiring and appliances.

Magnetic fields from electrical appliances typically fall off fairly rapidly at a rate somewhere between the inverse square (double the distance and you find one-quarter the fields) and the inverse cube (double the distance and you find one-eighth of the fields). Magnetic fields from wiring faults extend over much greater areas and fall off much more slowly.

Ground and basement floor rooms in cities usually have the highest magnetic fields from external underground cables and pipes and, in some cases, it will be difficult to achieve levels as low as 0.05 µT.

Average field levels

Average background magnetic fields in UK houses and similar buildings will generally be below 0.05 µT further than about a metre from most active appliances. Even an 8 kW electric shower should only produce about 0.05 µT at 1 metre away.

In blocks of flats, especially near the 'main service riser', the levels are likely to be higher than this, though they should generally still be below 0.10 µT.

The use of electric underfloor heating and 'off-peak' storage heaters will cause significantly higher levels when they are operating.

If your home is located within 100 metres of high-voltage over-head lines, your magnetic field exposure is likely to be higher – typically between 0.20 and 0.90 µT. About 5 per cent of homes at this kind of distance from high-voltage lines are likely to exceed 6 µT.

To help compare your home with the UK average, it is estimated that about 0.5 per cent of all homes in the UK have EMFs from external sources above 0.25 µT and the UK average background level from outside sources is about 0.0 4µT.

We believe that ideally, powerfrequency magnetic fields in the home should be less than 0.01 µT and electric fields should be less than 5 V/m. This is an extreme view, but in the majority of homes, levels of less than 0.03 µT and 10 V/m from *internal house sources* should be reasonably achievable in most of the places that people spend much time. We believe that these levels are OK for most people.

☺ There are suitable, reasonably priced, flexible screened cables now available, intended for eliminating electrical inter-ference in industrial and commercial use, which can be used instead of having the cables in metal pipes – provided the screens are carefully and effectively terminated. This is most suitable for rewiring an existing house which does not have the metal pipes in place.

☺ 'Automatic demand switches' eliminate electric fields from circuits that are not actually supplying power. These are useful as a remedial measure, but demand switches should not be needed in a well-designed new installation.

🗑 Powerfrequency magnetic fields will not be reduced by copper or lead sheeting. If the sheets are earthed, they will reduce electric fields.

🗑 Magnetic fields can only be effectively shielded using special steel sheeting. It is very difficult and expensive to shield large areas such as living or working spaces. It is always better to prevent the fields from being generated in the first place.

☺ Electric fields from an existing installation can be reduced by using special conductive paint (such as that from EMFields) on walls and ceilings, and on the floor underneath carpets, near wiring. You can decorate, or lay floor covering, on top of this earthed paint.

🗑 In 2005, the rules about who can legally carry out electrical work were tightened in the UK, under the Building Regulations, Part P requirements. Failure to comply with these regulations is a criminal offence, which could result in a maximum fine of £5,000 and/or imprisonment. Your house will probably need a Building Regulations Part P Inspection Certificate when you come to sell it.

Remember that electricity can be lethal, and all wiring installations should be checked to ensure that they are safe and that they fully comply with IEE regulations BS7671. This is not intended to keep electric and magnetic field levels down, although compliance with them will usually help to ensure low field levels. The suggestions made in this chapter can all be carried out within the requirements of the Institute of Electrical Engineers' wiring regulations (UK BS7671). (See Resources section for information available from Powerwatch on measuring EMFs and designing low EMF house wiring installations.)

In the Workplace

We've now looked at electropollution out and about, and at home. But workplaces can also expose you to significant levels of EMFs. Let's examine how.

Work can carry a high price these days. A 2004 UK Health and Safety Executive (HSE) report, quoting research published in 1981 by Sir Richard Doll and Sir Richard Peto,[26] suggests that the effect of occupation on cancer mortality accounted for between 2 and 8 per cent of total cancers. This would represent between 3,000 and 12,000 deaths from cancer that may occur every year in the UK as a result of occupational exposures to chemicals, radiation and possibly EMFs. The report states: 'Given the large numbers of people potentially exposed it is now recommended that non-ionising radiation (ie EMFs) be included in the list of priority agents that might cause leukaemia.' Note that this means adult leukaemia.

We believe that there is also evidence to support a possible link with breast cancer, brain cancer, prostate and testicular cancer.

Some industrial workers are exposed to high levels of electromagnetic fields – both at powerfrequency and radiofrequency. In

2008, the European and UK Physical Agents Directive will come fully into force. If you work near equipment that may give off this level of EMFs, we suggest that you ask your employer what they have done to check compliance with the new law.

Most occupational studies looking at jobs which are likely to have higher than usual EMF exposure have found a small to medium (for example, a doubling or more) increased incidence of leukaemias and brain cancers. A smaller, but significant, number of studies have associated occupational EMF exposure with breast cancer in women and prostate cancer in men.

We believe there is enough evidence to make it worth minimising your workplace EMF exposure. We have used the symbol '**??**' to indicate where there could be a problem, but not necessarily so. Further investigation is advised.

Offices and office equipment

Most offices contain an ever-increasing amount of electrical equipment, which contribute to EMFs and air pollution.

Our recommendations

Office equipment
Computers and **monitors (VDUs)** give off quite low levels of fields. For general use, see Chapter 4. In an office situation, people often spend more time at a computer monitor than they do in the home setting. Because of this, it is advisable to take the following precautions.

☺ To reduce the risk of developing eye strain (and repetitive strain injury), we advise that you take at least a five-minute break every hour.

☺ Make sure that the vertical refresh rate is set at 72 Hz at least, and preferably between 75 and 96 Hz. Windows sets the refresh rate at a default of 60 Hz, which some people might see as a slight flicker.

🗑 It is now illegal, in the UK and countries of the EC, for employers to allow workers to use a computer monitor with any visible instability in the display. Refresh frequencies at 100 Hz are reported to produce more headaches in users.

🗑 Many offices have quite a few VDUs in a relatively small space. All VDUs give off higher fields at the back and sides, so it is important to arrange office seating so that everyone sits at least a metre from the rear of a VDU. Ensure that the backs and sides of monitors are not next to places where people stop to exchange information, such as next to a drinks machine. Magnetic fields travel through walls, so watch the use of the next room.

☺ When a new computer monitor is bought, make sure that it is switched on (and fully running, not in 'standby energy saver' mode) in a well-ventilated room for about two weeks, because of the fire-retardant chemicals contained in the casings that will be released in the early stages of use.

🗑 LCD or TFT screens can emit significant levels of radio-frequency electric fields from the back illumination and scanning processes, and when run from the mains adapters they can give off very high electric fields next to the keyboard and display, as discussed in Chapter 4. If you feel your, or a colleague's, health is affected, measure the fields and take appropriate action (for example, first make sure each item is earthed).

☺ Since 1993, workers spending significant time on a computer have been entitled to a free eye test.

🗑 A survey by Dollond and Aitchison, Europe's largest optical group, found that over 70 per cent of people they spoke to were concerned that prolonged VDU work could affect their eyesight. Four out of every 10 who used computers stated that they had experienced sore eyes from staring at computer screens for too long.

☺ We blink about a third as often when using a computer compared with when we are talking to people. Use eye drops if your eyes feel dry. Humidity should ideally be 40 to 60 per cent.

🗑 **Photocopiers** give off quite high levels of EMFs from the motor. It would be advisable not to stand immediately next to the motor while it is working. Photocopiers also emit significant levels of ozone, and should always be in a well-ventilated room, or in a corridor. Volatile organic compounds (VOCs) are released, which increase with warmth, and double-sided copying. VOCs are given off even when the photocopier is not working, but is still switched on.

🗑 **Printers, scanners** and **fax machines** can all give off significant levels of EMFs near them, and some laser printers also release ozone. Keep chairs away from them and sit at least a half-metre away while they are working.

☺ Ink-jet printers are more ecologically friendly than laser printers and do not give off ozone.

🗑 Fluorescent **desk lights** (including the new energy-saver fluorescent lamps) require a transformer that generates EMFs.

☺ If you're using a small fluorescent lamp as a desk light, you may want to consider switching to an incandescent lamp, which generates virtually no EMFs.

?? The electric field from the motor of **desk fans** falls away rapidly; be at least half a metre away and make sure the cable leads away from you, as the electric fields from this are quite high.

?? All **cables** radiate electric fields. Keep wires tidy, in cable looms and as far from the body as possible.

🗑 🗑 🗑 We dealt with **DECT cordless phones** in detail in Chapter 3. We cannot recommend the use of DECT phones anywhere.

Air conditioning

Hot or cool air forced through the duct work of most **central heating and air conditioning systems** sets up friction that results in the loss of almost all the negative ions and also draws most of the positive ions out of the air as well. This air is then forced out through vents in to rooms, offices and passages – and as it passes through the vents more friction is set up that generates an additional overload of positive ions.

🗑 What finally comes out of most heating or air-conditioning outlets in offices is likely to be an overload of positive ions. An atmosphere high in positive ions is associated with dry throats, husky voices, headaches, and itchy or obstructed noses. For some people who are more sensitive, it has been found that the ability to breathe has been affected. Inadequately maintained central heating and air conditioning systems can result in a build-up of toxic particles which then get recirculated. It is often these systems which are responsible, among other things, for sick building syndrome. We also recommend that any air conditioning system passes air through active carbon filters that are checked and changed regularly.

☺ If you believe you may be affected, you might like to see whether a good negative ioniser will help improve the air quality. For a supplier of good negative ionisers, see the Resources section.

Reducing exposure in the office

DO

✔ Take at least a five-minute break every hour, when you are using a computer. Move around during this time.

✔ Sit at least 50 cm from the front and more than 1 metre from the rear of a VDU. Check any 'leisure' space for proximity to VDUs.

✔ Ensure that a new computer monitor is properly 'run in' in a well-ventilated room for about two weeks before use to get rid of the worst of the volatile organic compounds.

✔ Check electric field levels from an LCD or TFT screen monitor. Earth if necessary.

✔ Have a free eye test if you feel you are being affected. Use eye drops if your eyes feel dry.

✔ Make sure that windows are sideways to the computer screen, so there are no reflections in the screen and no times of the day when it is too bright behind the screen.

✔ Ensure that the resolution, brightness and contrast of the screen are optimally adjusted for you so that you can easily read all the information on the VDU screen without straining. It is worth experimenting with changing these.

✔ Make sure there are no reflections on the screen from overhead lights, windows or desk lamps.

- ✔ If possible, keep at least a metre away from working electrical appliances.
- ✔ Ensure photocopiers are in a well-ventilated room or corridor. Install an extractor fan near the photocopier if there is no air conditioning.
- ✔ Use an ink-jet printer in preference to a laser printer.
- ✔ Keep any fans at a reasonable distance from you.
- ✔ Ensure that central heating or air conditioning systems are regularly maintained.
- ✔ Ensure you have good natural ventilation and natural light wherever possible.
- ✔ Try a negative air ioniser to improve the atmosphere.

DON'T

- ✗ Don't stand or sit close to working electrical equipment.
- ✗ Use a fluorescent desk lamp with care.
- ✗ Don't have a digital cordless phone on the desk.
- ✗ Don't run electric wires under desks close to your feet or legs.

Schools and colleges

School secretaries obviously work in offices, and will have the same sort of exposure we saw above. School labs are unlikely to have the same sort of sophisticated equipment as other research labs, but if you are unsure about EMFs, it may be worth checking them. It could make a good GCSE project.

Our recommendations

🗑 🗑 School libraries and IT facilities may have wireless local area networked (wLAN) computers. These can give a high background level of microwaves to which teachers and pupils will be exposed for most of the day. We are against every pupil having a wireless enabled laptop computer on which they do all their school work. This is because 20 or more laptops and a wireless access point fill the classroom with several volts per metre of pulsing microwave radiation electrosmog. Electrically sensitive children will react very badly to this exposure, which is associated with memory and concentration problems and increased aggressive behaviour.

☺ Laptops wired by Ethernet using standard cables are fine. The pupils can use their laptops on their own for most work and plug in a network cable when they need to access files on the school server computer or on the internet. Infrared data connections are also believed to be safe.

🗑 Some interactive whiteboards, used to display computer and video images in the classroom also use microwave technology. The whiteboard display (using back or front projection) should be connected by wire to the teacher's controller PC and will not then be a problem. However, some are now being sold with built-in wireless networks to connect to the teacher's PC and to wireless connected interactive pen displays that can be moved around the classroom and operated by pupils. These wireless options will increase the ambient level of electrosmog in the classroom.

Hospitals and clinics

Ironically, some of the high-tech equipment now used in medicine can contribute to ill health.

Our recommendations

General

☺ There is a wide and diverse range of medical devices that emit EMFs in one form or another. Generally, the use of these is beneficial to the patient.

🗑 However, we would choose to avoid any unnecessary exposure that is not specifically needed for a clinical decision. In other words, no 'routine' X-rays or ultrasound scans and the like. That reduces the exposure of both professional staff and patients.

🗑 It is accepted that about 0.6 per cent of UK cancers are due to medical X-ray procedures. It is not known how many radiographers are affected.

Computerised (Axial) Tomography (CT or CAT) scans have been used increasingly in the past two decades, both in the UK and the USA. By their nature, CAT scans result in a significantly higher patient radiation dose than conventional X-ray examinations. One abdominal CAT scan can increase the risk of a fatal cancer by 1 in 2000 according to the US Food and Drug Administration.[27]

There has been a very concerning rise in the use of CAT scans of children in the USA. Recent studies show that 600,000 abdominal and head CAT examinations annually in children under 15 years of age could result in 500 deaths from cancer due to CAT radiation.[28]

We suggest that you ask your doctor about the clinical advantages of any suggested CAT scan and, if a scan is really necessary, why a safer MRI scan could not be used instead.

?? As long as the radiographers are in properly screened areas it is unlikely that they will receive much of a dose.

?? Some of the electrical control gear used in hospitals can give off significant levels of powerfrequency magnetic fields due to the power being used. If you are concerned, you need to get the field levels measured to see which areas you should avoid.

Fluorescent lights are generally used to light hospitals. We discussed this kind of lighting in Chapter 4.

🗑 Fluorescent lights can affect people with EHS quite badly. Some of the early (circa.1975–1985) high-frequency (low flicker) fluorescent light fittings gave off high levels of radiofrequency noise in the 35 kHz to 150 kHz frequency range. These can produce headaches and flu-like symptoms in workers.

☺ Lift control gear and motors are usually on the roof or in the basement and so are well out of the way of staff and patients.

?? Maintenance workers need to be aware of the high magnetic fields in restricted areas.

Most modern hospitals contain a large amount of specialised machinery for diagnostic and treatment purposes. Some of this equipment will give off very high EMFs for the patient, for whom the benefits are likely to outweigh the risks.

?? Staff working with the equipment on a daily basis may have less than adequate protection. It is assumed that all workers are fully healthy with a strong immune system and the protection they require is less than that of the patients. On the whole this assumption is correct, but not always and, of course, staff have much longer and more regular exposure.

As the health effects from high exposures may be cumulative, it is important that you are very careful when working round such equipment.

A consultant anaesthetist, Richard, had to take early retirement as he had developed severe electrical hypersensitivity. Unfortunately, he received a very bad response from his professional medical colleagues who put it down to undiagnosed psychiatric problems and suggested that he take medication to lower his stress levels. When he is away from electrical equipment his health is much better.

Diathermy equipment used by some physiotherapists probably causes the highest occupational EMF exposures. These use high-powered radiofrequency radiation to heat body tissue. This is not well contained, and the treatment room as a whole can be permeated with significant levels of energy. Miscarriages and congenital malformations in children born to physiotherapists using diathermy equipment have been reported in several studies.[29] As a result of this, we would recommend that everyone using such equipment should have the RF field levels measured, paying attention to the places with highest readings so that they can avoid these.

Magnetic resonance imaging (MRI) scanners expose people to high levels of magnetic fields.

Some cases of EHS have been triggered by an MRI scan.

In 2008, as we've seen, the Physical Agents Directive will reduce the safety limit for operating staff exposure. It is necessary for staff to be exposed to significant levels of EMFs and X-rays when operating equipment such as MRI and CAT scanners. This may cause employment problems and some units may have to close.

☺ **EEG/EKG/ECG** equipment will not normally expose you to significant EMFs.

Dental surgeries
☺ Dental surgeries do not generally have high sources of EMF.

🗑 Small X-ray machines should be used with care.

Laboratories
?? Most laboratories contain many pieces of electronic equipment. It is a good idea to try and keep at least 50 cm between you and any equipment (especially power supplies or high-voltage equipment), though this isn't always possible. If you are concerned about your EMF exposure in a laboratory, then you really need to measure both the powerfrequency and microwave field levels.

Hairdressing salons

There are generally two kinds of **hairdryers** used in salons: a hood under which customers sit, and handheld dryers for blow-dry styling.

Our recommendations

🗑 Both types of dryer give off high levels of EMFs. Pregnant hairdressers should be careful where they hold handheld dryers and limit the number of times they are used in a day. Hood hair-dryers can produce high magnetic fields. Hair stylists and hairdressers should try to keep their distance from them, especially if pregnant, or if they have a compromised immune system.

Shops

Anti-theft security systems, barcode readers and the like are increasingly features of high-street shops. Here's what to look out for.

Our recommendations

🗑 **Electronic tills** are now the norm in most shops – and they can be problematic. People with EHS may have problems operating the tills, or even just standing near them. Some tills communicate with the main stock control and accounting computers using microwaves.

☺ **Bar code readers** use a scanning infrared beam to read the lines and do not present a problem.

🗑 If you are sensitive to radiofrequency radiation then you may find **Radio Frequency Identification (RFID)** tags a problem. These tags are now being used by many large stores as a means of stock control. RFID tags send out a code when they are 'interrogated' by a special scanner. These emit strong EMFs to transfer the power into the passive RFID tag, in turn enabling it to transmit its code back to the scanner.

The handheld units may be particularly problematic. Some designs can even be strapped on the worker's arm so that they can have their hands free.

🗑 🗑 Some **scanners** for RFID tags, and for more basic security tags, use low-frequency RF fields (tens to hundreds of kHz), such as the large vertical coils that you pass through at the exits to many supermarkets. The exposures that you receive from these can be very high indeed. Store workers should not stand close to these coils.

🗑 Increasingly, RFID tags are being energised by a microwave beam – either at the checkout or in a handheld stock-control scanner unit. There is even an experimental system under-going trials that would be built into the shelves where expensive items are held.

🗑 Another system undergoing field trials has electronic receivers that display price labels for the shelves that are regularly updated by microwave signals transmitted by the stock-control computer.

All these things increase the electrosmog levels in our shops, and may make it impossible for EHS people to work in them.

☺ **Fridges and freezers,** especially in specialist freezer shops where there are lots of them, give off high levels of EMFs near to the motors, but these are usually in the base and not close to people.

Internet and broadband cafes

Our recommendations

🗑 As these now house wireless 'hotspot' access points for laptop computers there will probably be quite high background levels of radiofrequency radiation nearby. You should avoid working in them if you are sensitive to such radiation.

Libraries

The magnetic security equipment that logs the books and other loans in and out of a library can emit very high levels of magnetic fields.

Our recommendations

🗑 It is unlikely to be a problem for library users, unless they have EHS, but we have seen units built into the work surfaces that expose library staff to very high levels of EMFs while they are operating the equipment.

◻ You should be especially careful if pregnant, as this equipment is often placed at the height that will expose the growing baby to high fields that could be hazardous.

Fire and police stations

Our recommendations

The **practice towers** in the grounds of **fire stations** are frequently used for locating mobile phone base stations.

◻ The crew and support staff occupying the buildings surrounding the tower may be exposed to high levels of radio-frequency electrosmog. There will be hotspots on the tower which the crew will be intermittently exposed to, and to which some may react.

◻ A more important safety issue for firemen concerns mobile phone base station antennas mounted on the sides of buildings, including high blocks of flats. These are not always very noticeable and are hardly ever labelled as emitting microwave radiation. It is easy to exceed the high ICNIRP exposure guidance levels within a few metres of the front of such antennas. They should be clearly labelled with yellow and black RF Radiation Hazard warning triangles, but there is as yet no requirement under UK or EC law to do this.

Police stations may often have TETRA masts on top of the building. This is the emergency services digital system which replaced the analogue police radio system. TETRA is a private radio communications system that is different from the public mobile telephone networks. There is an ongoing scientific debate about whether this difference produces more adverse health effects than ordinary masts.

🗑 TETRA masts are usually lower power than ordinary mobile phone masts, but some people are reporting high levels of adverse health effects when near TETRA masts. Because TETRA operates at a lower transmission frequency the radiation penetrates people and buildings more easily than ordinary phone mast radiation.

🗑 Police who use the handsets have apparently been reporting high levels of sickness, including cancers of the oesophagus (where some of the handsets are carried on operational duty). TETRA radiation seems to be more biologically active than GSM signals. The handsets, but not the masts, pulse strongly at 17.6 Hz, which is a brainwave frequency and has also been shown to affect the way minerals and nutrients pass through cell membranes, reducing the health of the cells.[30]

Petrol stations

Apart from electronic tills (see 'Shops', page 139), some petrol stations have mobile phone base stations in the price signs.

Our recommendations

?? They should not affect the sales people any more than other mobile phone masts, though they can be quite near staff working in the retail part of the site. Petrol and exhaust fumes are probably a much greater hazard, as some substances in them are carcinogenic.

Electricity and telecommunication industries

Our recommendations

?? Most workers in these industries are likely to have at least intermittent quite high occupational exposures to EMFs. They will receive what is considered to be adequate training in appropriate precautionary measures, however.

☺ Some maintenance personnel have chosen to carry EMF monitors to measure their own exposure, as they are not entirely sure whether their health is being fully protected by current guidelines.

🗑 In 1994, Dr Gilles Thériault reported a very strong association between various cancers and abrupt changes in levels of EMF exposure from electric powerlines and equipment. Previously just the average 50 or 60 Hz EMF exposure levels were measured, but the work by Thériault and others showed that electrical spikes up to several thousand hertz may be more hazardous.[31] This created a political and commercial backlash and the work has not been adequately followed up.

Factories and warehouses

Our recommendations

?? Many industrial machines and processes expose workers to high EMF levels – both powerfrequency and radiofrequency. These are undergoing scrutiny as the 2008 date for the implementation of the European and UK Physical Agents Directive approaches. Many workers' exposures are believed to currently be above the proposed new legal maximum levels.

?? We know of places where levels regularly exceed the new guidance. These include **power stations, steel works, induction and arc furnaces, marine engineering works, induction heaters in chemical works, plasma etching and torch facilities, RF metal sputtering facilities, and permanent magnet makers**. These are only a few and there are obviously others that we don't know about. If you work in one of these heavy industries, you may like to have the work place assessed. Sometimes easy changes to working practice can significantly reduce your daily exposure to EMFs.

▥ Cancer is not the only outcome. Higher incidence of children with congenital malformations born to high-voltage **switchyard workers** in Sweden were traced to chromosome changes in sperm, probably arising from EMF exposure.[32]

▥ **Welders** are exposed to very high magnetic fields that can easily exceed ICNIRP guidance levels, often in combination with air pollutants.

▥ **Electric forklift truck drivers** are often sitting directly over the batteries and electrical cables and can have very high transient magnetic fields in their lower-trunk and genital areas. Cases of testicular cancer and infertility have been reported, but we can find no comprehensive study to confirm that this is a general problem.

▥ People using **electric industrial sewing machines** are exposed to very high magnetic fields from the motors. Some machines, with two-core mains cables, will also give off high electric fields. Ensure that you keep your body as far away as possible from the motor.

In 1994, Dr Gene Sobel of the University of Southern California reported a strong association between EMFs and Alzheimer's disease. The study concentrated on sewing machinists. Despite very limited funding, Sobel continued to build on his original finding and, in 1996, a Swedish researcher, Maria Feychting, reported some support for the EMF–Alzheimer's link.

Recording and TV studios

Our recommendations

?? There are high powerfrequency magnetic fields near lighting cables and the power control units, though the actual lighting desks are usually fine. The highest source, the bulk-tape demagnetiser or eraser, has almost disappeared because everything has gone digital and computerised. Until now, the fields near these erasers could be extremely high, exceeding ICNIRP guidance levels.

?? Studio radio talk-back systems can produce quite high RF levels depending on the type and how the installation has been made. We recently heard of one where levels in a corridor exceeded public ICNIRP levels. The system was changed to correct this, and confirms the need for workers to request formal safety tests to be made.

?? The RF fields near the transmitter dish antennas on outside broadcast vans can be very high.

Transport

Our recommendations

🗑 Some 10 to 25 per cent of UK train drivers report 'missing time', in which they were unaware of their surroundings. However brief this 'absence' may be, if it is at a critical place, such as coming up to a red light, it could lead to fatal accidents. It may be that train drivers who have these sorts of episodes have a degree of EHS, as intermittently they are subject to high levels of EMFs. Diesel-electric trains produce EMFs very close to the engines.

🗑 Drivers of local suburban trains, underground trains and trams are also subject to high levels of EMFs. These types of transport use 'pseudo-DC (direct current)' with a large AC (alternating current) component – it's known as 'full wave rectified unsmoothed AC'. This gives rise to *very* high DC and AC fields at floor level due to the underfloor traction equipment. No research has been done into these fields recently, as train operators have concerned themselves with other health and safety issues which have taken priority.

However, it can clearly be imagined that EHS drivers may make less than optimal decisions when in charge of these vehicles.

If you feel that you or your work colleagues may be affected by EMF exposure, measure the fields. If they are high, negotiate a change in the working environment wherever possible.

6

Out and About

So far, we have looked mainly at relatively long-term exposure to EMFs, such as in bedrooms or offices, and what to do to prevent or halt it. But what about those times when we dip into and out of EMFs?

We are, after all, exposed to EMFs while we are travelling and visiting friends, shopping, pubbing & clubbing, going to clinics or hospitals and a myriad other places. In doing all this, we are just paying relatively fleeting visits to the workplaces of others. For instance, I travel in a train – which is the train driver's workplace, so he or she and I may well be exposed to different levels of EMF. Because of this, there is some overlap between Chapter 5 and this chapter, and depending on the circumstances of your work and other activities, you may want to read these two chapters together.

Should you worry about this shifting, intermittent exposure, or just get on with living your life? Only you can decide, but we believe it does matter. You should enjoy life and that will mean taking risks, but you should also be able to decide what risks are worth taking. It is much like the sort of personal cost/benefit analysis that seems so popular with businesses and government today.

Railways

We read in Chapter 2 that many UK railway lines are electrified. The power reaches the engines by means of overhead lines, or a third rail running parallel to the two rails the train runs on. Both systems create high magnetic fields for rail travellers.

Peak level exposure of 1.6 microtesla or more have been associated with more than double the risk of miscarriage.[33] Electric trains commonly expose people to transient levels way above this, and in certain seats (see below), levels can rise to well over 100 microtesla.

Our recommendations

▤ The **high magnetic fields** in some electrified trains can make journeys both uncomfortable for people with EHS, and potentially dangerous for all pregnant women, especially in the early stages of pregnancy.

▤ **Trains with overhead wires** are usually powered at 25,000 volts AC and produce a significant electric field over 100 V/m inside by the windows.

▤ In these trains, carriages that have pantographs (roof-mounted 'pickup' arms) have **pillars** inside, where power from the overhead lines is brought down to the motors. There are usually two pillars in these carriages, and they can produce very high EMFs, often next to seats.

It is probably best to sit away from the window seats, where electric fields are higher than in seats nearer the middle of the train.

?? Underfloor motors and ventilation equipment also produce high EMFs. It is worth finding a seat which is not in a place with high fields. The only real way to do this is to carry a powerfrequency magnetic field monitor with you.

🗑 Tsuyoshi Hondou, a physicist at Tohuku University in Japan, reported in 2002 that lots of people using mobile phones inside a train carriage could exceed international safety limits for microwave exposure, because microwaves bounce back from the carriage's metal structure. He believes this could have serious health risks for other passengers.[34] Hondou also suggested that the problem might apply to buses.

🗑 British Rail are experimenting with making mobile phone signals available in railway tunnels, a move that will expose travellers to more background radiation. Passengers with EHS may already be aware of the sudden 'logging on' of phones on standby as they seek a base station on emerging from a tunnel.

🗑 Some train operators are now wiring their carriages for 'WiFi', so that laptop users can use broadband internet services while they are travelling. Wireless internet facilities are also being installed in many train stations. These increase every traveller's microwave exposure.

🗑 The UK Department for Transport reported in November 2005 that **body scanners** using high-tech millimetre wave (tera-hertz) imaging technology that can see through clothes and detect bombs and weapons are among the technology being tested to boost security on the UK rail network. The first trials will be on the London Paddington to Heathrow Express service. There will be a body scanner for people, and their luggage will also be X-rayed.

If the system works, it will then be rolled out across all major rail and tube stations. King's Cross and Euston are next in line. Health implications are unknown, but this is exposing people to another new form of electromagnetic energy that penetrates their bodies.

🗑 Suburban trains, underground trains and trams have *very* high DC and AC fields, pulsing 100 (or 120) times every second at floor level because of the underfloor traction equipment. They also produce transient surges every time they start moving. These are suspected of being very biologically active and potentially harmful, for pregnant women in particular.

Underground trains

Our recommendations

?? Most underground trains use DC electricity (like a battery), but still pulses at 100 or 120 Hz. Some underground train carriages may expose you to higher magnetic fields than even the official ICNIRP safety guidance levels (in our opinion, definitely not good news for pregnant women).

🗑 Mobile phone operators are experimenting with installing equipment that will enable the phones to be used in underground trains. This may make the situation much harder for people with EMF sensitivities to travel as many people will use their mobile phones in a confined space, irradiating fellow passengers.

Trams

Electric tram systems produce high magnetic fields from the electricity used to power the motors. Anybody sitting above the motors will be exposed to high fields, as magnetic fields can travel through the floor of the tram. As tram designs vary you will need to use an EMF meter to identify where the high EMFs are.

Our recommendations

?? Be aware of where the power take-up units are and sit as far as possible from them if you are pregnant, have children with you or have a poor immune system. Ideally, use an EMF meter to find the seats with the lowest exposure.

🗑 Changes in magnetic fields such as those caused every time the tram starts and accelerates have been linked to an increased risk of miscarriage, especially in the first three months of pregnancy (see Chapter 7).

Planes and airports

Certain changes in the pipeline, such as the installation of mobile phone and wireless technology, are going to make plane travel virtually impossible for people with EHS.

Our recommendations

🗑 The personal lights above the seats in a plane are often high-frequency fluorescent lights and can be sources of significant electric fields. Turn yours off.

🗑 Some planes have in-flight video screens built into the back of each seat. These are a source of high-frequency fields both for the people watching the screen and for those whose seat it is fitted into.

🗑 Airbus and American Airlines are intending to make inflight mobile phone technology available. They are installing a pico-cell base station – effectively, a small mobile phone mast –

onboard the aircraft. (See Chapter 3 for an overview of the risks posed by mobile phone masts.)

🗑 Boeing is to install wireless computer technology on aircraft, and Airbus has also trialled several wireless network technologies such as Bluetooth, Wi-Fi and wideband CDMA.

🗑 Metal and X-ray detectors are used in airports for security checks. People with EHS may well react to these scans and workers may be exposed to quite high levels of EMFs.

🗑 Whole-body scanners which use frequencies in the terahertz (THz) part of the EMF spectrum are increasingly used, as they can reveal the presence of non-metal weaponry.

A consortium of European universities reported on research carried out between 2001 and 2004 on terahertz radiation.[35] They concluded that 'there are indications that THz radiation could induce damages on a molecular scale in certain biological systems due to the mechanism of resonant absorption'.

Airport authorities may have undertaken cost/benefit analyses that show the risk from terrorists as greater than the risk of harm from terahertz radiation. But it still seems premature to us to use this kind of EMF radiation on the travelling public and airport personnel, when adverse health effects are possible although still unclear.

Car, buses and coaches

Cars, especially the newer models that sport a number of high-tech features, can be surprisingly high in EMFs. Remember that fields of 0.4 microtesla have been associated with ill health (see page 24), yet measurements in some cars far exceed that.

For drivers with EHS, driving can be dangerous: exposure to high EMFs can result in loss of co-ordination and fatigue that may lead to dangerous errors. As you will see below, the best insurance is to buy older, less high-tech car models and limit your exposure – walking more is great for your health, in any case!

Our recommendations

?? There are several potential sources of high EMFs in cars. Cars have electrical and electronic equipment (power wiring, fan motors, computerised controls and dashboards) that can disturb electrically sensitive people. The front seat can be a particular risk area: a friend measured 13 microtesla in a small hotspot in her Honda, a level over 30 times higher than that associated with increased risk of childhood leukaemia.

In February 2002, Volvo models V70, S60 and S80 had measured EMFs of 12 to 18 microtesla in the driver's part of the car. The three models in question have the battery in the boot and only a single power cable to the engine at the front. Such wiring always results in high EMFs.

Volvo did not dispute the findings, although Ford (which owns Volvo) initially made the following statement: 'Because there is no evidence about risks of electromagnetic fields in cars, Volvo is not currently taking technical or other measures.' Yet the sales of Volvo cars dipped after this was made public.

Since then, Volvo has developed a 'fix' for concerned owners, but they have not actively marketed it. Some other cars (such as BMW and Mercedes) also carry their batteries in the rear and display similar problems.

🗑 Some upmarket cars such as Jaguars, Mercedes and BMWs have electronic control units under (or even as a part of) the driver's seat. These will give off high magnetic fields.

?? Also worth checking is whether the angle and position of car seats are electrically controlled. These have higher EMFs than mechanically operated seats.

Choose your car carefully, preferably using a meter (see Resources) to detect the fields, and keep journeys as short as practicable in cars when you are unaware of the field levels you may be exposed to.

> **Peter, who has EHS, has chosen a car because it is very simple – an old convertible with few electronic 'gadgets'. He can remove the door windows, soft top, and even fold down the windscreen if he begins to feel uncomfortable. When using the heater, he finds he needs to have it blowing at his feet and also needs to open the windows to avoid exhaustion.**
>
> **Jenny bought a new BMW X5 in 2002, but found fields of 8 microtesla in the car. She felt quite ill whenever she travelled in it, but had not had problems in the previous car used by the family. She felt worse when the car was stationary with the engine idling.**

🗑 The steel reinforcing of radial tyres is often magnetised during manufacture. As the tyres rotate, they produce low-frequency pulsing EMFs that some people react adversely to so, if you are sensitive, it is advisable to have your tyres and wheels de-magnetised (degaussed), although there are few firms offering this service. Otherwise, it is best to sit in the front passenger seat and choose a traditional car as some 'people carriers' have the front wheels very close to the front seats.

Cars can have high levels of EMFs due to this problem with the tyres, the wiring from the battery to the alternator charger and also high microwave levels because of the different Bluetooth devices now being fitted as standard. An anti-static strip (which prevents the build up of static electricity in a car) is unlikely to help, unless one of your regular symptoms is electric shocks.

☺ As a general rule, the older and cheaper the model of car, the better it is in EMF terms.

🗑 It is advisable not to sit in seats directly above the wheels on buses or coaches, for the same reason as cars.

How to limit your exposure in vehicles

DO

- ✔ Carry a meter to help you choose the seat with lowest EMF fields in all public vehicles: trains, underground trains, trams, buses and coaches.
- ✔ If possible, sit in a carriage where the use of mobile phones is not allowed.
- ✔ Carry a meter to help you choose a car. Most new cars may have high microwave readings as well as low-frequency EMFs.
- ✔ Switch off your personal light in a plane.
- ✔ Do not watch in-flight entertainment. Be aware that if the person behind you is using theirs, you too will be exposed to high EMFs. Choose a

flight from an airline offering basic rather than luxury options if you have EHS.

✔ If you feel unwell in the passenger side of a car, try sitting in the back, where the field exposures could be lower.

✔ Keep your journeys as short as practicable in cars you're not familiar with. Check with a meter for the seat with the lowest EMF exposure.

DON'T

✘ Don't stand near scanning machinery in an airport.

✘ Don't sit immediately above the wheels in buses and coaches.

✘ Don't buy a car with lots of electronic gadgets. These have the highest EMF levels.

Controlled entrance/exit bars

Some housing associations, factories, office buildings and the like have installed security systems to restrict access to the site. RFID (standing for 'radio frequency identification device') systems use EMFs to energise an identity tag carried by authorised people. That then sends a radiofrequency signal back to confirm the user's identity.

Our recommendations

🗑 These systems are likely to cause problems for people with EHS.

☺ Swipe card and bar code systems should be fine.

🗑 There are now experimental RFID tag activators designed to track cars and other vehicles entering and leaving 'toll road' areas. One type is suspended on wires high across the road. If you were to stand directly underneath, this type could expose you to levels that exceed the current official EMF safety levels.

Mobile phone masts

Chapter 2 contains detailed information about these masts. You will be unable to avoid them when you are out and about because, although they're not always visible, they are now very widespread.

They may be part of the street furniture, or an unobtrusive fixture in a shopping centre. They may be wall-mounted or placed on equipment such as lampposts or CCTV equipment. Most mobile phone operators keep the power levels reasonably low, though it is quite variable. Some produce high radio-frequency radiation close to the mast.

Some are being placed in the foyers of airports, hotels, GPs' surgeries, coffee shops, student halls of residence and schools so individuals can use their phones with the minimum of fuss.

They are likely to present a problem for people with EHS.

Shops

As we saw in the last chapter, shops are now full of high-tech devices that can present a problem for people with electrical sensitivity.

Our recommendations

🗑 🗑 **Security tagging devices** that look for tags that are then deactivated at the checkout can expose you to high radio-frequency fields. Scientists at the University of Utah[36] reported that anti-theft security tagging, the mechanism of which is usually sited in pillars close to shop doors, could be exposing children under five years old to twice the EMF safety limits. Presumably this conclusion was reached when taking into account children's average height and body weight. For people with EHS, this could also have a significant effect. Although the fields are localised and transitory, they are pulsed – which as we have seen is believed to be biologically active. Occasionally, they are placed so that a customer has to spend some time exposed to this field level while their purchases are dealt with.

?? Most shops have **electronic tills** at the checkout. People who have EHS may have problems standing near them. Some now 'communicate' with the main stock control and accounting computers using microwaves, which will add to your exposure.

☺ **Barcode readers** use a scanning infrared beam to read the lines and do not usually present a problem.

🗑 **Radio frequency identification or RFID** tags are now being used by many large department stores as a means of stock control, especially for more costly items. RFID tags send out a code when they are 'interrogated' by a special scanner. These emit a strong EMF to transfer the power into the passive RFID tag, which enables it to transmit its code back to the scanner. If you are sensitive to radiofrequency radiation, then you may find these a problem.

🗑 Increasingly, RFID tags are energised by a microwave beam – either at the checkout or in a handheld stock-control scanner unit. There is even an experimental system undergoing trials that is designed to be built into the shelves where expensive items are held.

🗑 Another system now being tested has electronic receivers that display price labels for the shelves that are regularly updated by microwave signals transmitted by the stock-control computer.

All these things significantly boost electrosmog.

Internet and broadband cafes

Our recommendations

?? As these usually house a wireless 'hotspot' access point for laptop computers and the like, there are likely to be quite high background levels of radiofrequency radiation nearby. You should avoid them if you are sensitive to it.

Hairdressing salons

Our recommendations

🗑 Hood-style hairdryers produce a very high EMF. There is usually more than one heat setting, and the fields will be higher as the heat is greater, though most are produced by the motor. Sitting still under the hood regularly may have an adverse effect on some people, although intermittent or infrequent exposure is unlikely to affect most. Any metal in hairpins or curlers will increase the effect.

Hospitals, clinics and surgeries

In Chapter 5 we looked at some of the hospital and clinic equipment exposing workers to potentially high levels of EMFs. Here is what you can expect if you're a visitor or patient.

Today's hospitals are full of electric and electronic components, including intensive care units with life-support systems, operating theatres, MRI scanners, autoclaving machines, floor polishers and other types of equipment almost too numerous to mention. So in-patients, out-patients and visitors will all be subjected to a cocktail of different kinds of exposure.

There is no answer to reducing exposure generally. It is always a question of whether the need for medical knowledge, accurate diagnosis and effective treatment of the individual concerned offsets the potential damage that can be caused by EMF exposure. If you suffer from EHS, going into hospital as a patient or visitor can, however, be a harrowing experience.

Our recommendations

?? Hospitals are usually lit with fluorescent lights, which we discussed in Chapter 4. These can affect people with EHS quite badly.

?? We believe it is worth giving very serious consideration to whether you wish to expose yourself to 'routine' **X-rays**. A study published in *The Lancet* that investigated the risk of developing cancer from exposure to medical X-ray tests has estimated that 0.6 per cent of all cancers diagnosed in the UK are caused by medical X-rays.[37] According to the researchers, this would account for roughly 700 of the 124,000 new cases of cancer in the UK each year.

?? You may like to consider the advisability of regular **mammograms** over just regular physical breast examinations. Mammograms do diagnose possible breast cancers a couple of years earlier than physical exams, but the evidence is decidedly mixed as to whether the survival rate among women diagnosed by mammogram is any better that those who did not have a mammogram. The dose from each mammogram is about sevenfold higher than you would receive from a normal chest X-ray.

?? If you are pregnant, you may want to consider carefully whether you want to expose your unborn child to **ultrasound scans**. The increasing practice of vaginal ultrasound may have more health effects, as the foetus is smaller and the exposure higher.

A UK survey showed that, for 1 in 200 babies where the pregnancy was terminated because the ultrasound showed major abnormalities, the diagnosis on post-mortem was less severe than predicted by ultrasound and the termination was probably unjustified (see Appendix).

A summary of the safety of ultrasound in human studies published in May 2002 concluded that 'there may be a relation between prenatal ultrasound exposure and adverse outcome. Some of the reported effects include growth restriction, delayed speech, dyslexia, and non-right-handedness (which can be seen as a marker of damage to the developing brain) associated with ultrasound exposure.' Other effects that have been reported are damage to the myelin that covers nerves, and the irreversible loss of brain cells [see Buckley in Further Reading]. Even official agencies are starting to be concerned about foetal ultrasound scans. We suggest that you try to minimise them for your child's sake.

🗑 **Computer aided tomography** (CAT or CT) has been used increasingly in the past two decades. The National Radiological Protection Board (now part of the Health Protection Agency), reported that in 1998, CAT scans constituted 4 per cent of all medical examinations, contributing 40 per cent of the collective effective dose of X-rays.

The cost of buying and running CAT scanners is much less than for MRI systems (see below), so hospitals often ask doctors to use them where possible. The use of paediatric CAT examinations has been increasing at a still faster rate since helical CAT scanners reduced the exposure time from around 1 minute to 1 second, eliminating the need for anaesthesia.

CAT scans give a significantly higher dose of radiation (between forty and a hundred times higher) than a conventional X-ray examination. In terms of dose, CAT scans now probably represent the largest source of radiation exposure from diagnostic examinations, both in the US and the UK. We believe that MRI scans are much safer than CAT scans as they do not expose the patient to X-rays, and we do not generally recommend CAT scans for children.

?? **Magnetic resonance imaging** (MRI) scanners use strong magnetic fields and radiofrequency fields to build up a picture of the inside of the body. Despite this, they are probably the safest form of imaging, and about a million MRI scans are performed each year in the UK.

Stronger magnetic fields provide higher resolution images. Some people say that MRI scans have triggered their EHS. Side effects can arise from the compound injected into the patient, known as gadolinium contrast agent, which accumulates in scar tissue, tumours and the like so they become easier to see during the scan. In any case, people with EHS are unlikely to be able to tolerate the high EMFs used. We suggest that you think carefully about whether the benefits are likely to outweigh any possible disadvantages.

☺ **EEG/EKG/ECG** equipment will not normally expose you to significant EMFs.

☺ **TENS** (transcutaneous electrical nerve stimulator) units can help to exercise and relax muscles, using electrical stimulation to give rise to natural endorphins that can give pain relief. Although the pulsing electric fields are having a clear biological effect, the scientific literature does not provide any reason to consider these to be hazardous from an EMF point of view.

?? Diathermy equipment employing radiofrequency radiation probably causes the highest EMF exposures. Some physiotherapists use diathermy units to treat patients with rheumatic disorders of the joints and muscles, inflammatory disorders of the respiratory organs, the kidneys and urinary tracts, and all disorders resulting from poor circulation.

The radiofrequency radiation from this equipment penetrates deep into body tissues to stimulate blood flow and to heat the treated area. The RF field can be continuous or pulsed depending on the application. A timer is often used to control the length of treatment.

The units can use frequencies of 27, 434, 915, and 2450 MHz, and some can emit 900 watts – which will heat body tissue by many degrees Celsius. The heating effect on parts of the body that have been exposed to RF radiation may last up to 90 minutes and increase tissue temperature significantly. We do not know whether there are adverse health effects from receiving diathermy treatments, although people with EHS may well be affected.

?? Many hospitals provide **Patientline** – bedside entertainment units that offer TV and telephone, radio, electronic games and films. These give off measurable levels of EMFs which may affect patients who are bedbound for significant lengths of time, and whose immune systems may already be compromised. Visitors staying an hour or two at a time are unlikely to be affected.

?? Certain **implanted medical devices**, including insulin delivery systems and pacemakers, are also sensitive to environmental AC magnetic fields.

People using homeopathic remedies should take routine precautions when storing them. These are easily de-potentised by high magnetic fields, so the environment needs to be carefully monitored. Homeopathic hospitals should take great care in manufacturing (especially if the sucussing is done using machines generating EMFs) and storing the finished remedies.

Hospitals and doctors' surgeries that have special units for patients with EHS – which are very rare indeed – should take a sensitive approach to the presence of equipment and lighting to accommodate patients' special requirements.

🗑 **Doctors' surgeries** generally have quite high EMF levels from internal wiring and equipment. An EMF meter will help you find the best place to sit.

🗑 **Dental surgeries** present a more complex picture. On the one hand, they are not generally high sources of EMF. They do, however, rely heavily on fluorescent lighting for good visibility (see page 99 for information on this kind of lighting). The halogen lights commonly used in practices are basically bright filament lights and should not be a problem as long as the transformer is some distance from the patient.

Of more concern are the small **X-ray machines** used in dental practices. Occasional X-rays, used for diagnostic purposes when there may be a problem, are fine. However, all X-rays slightly increase the risk of cancer and we do not recommend them unless you suspect an existing problem that needs further investigation. We don't advise them for routine health checks.

🗑 Dr Keith Baverstock of the University of Kuopio, Finland, who has worked for the UK Medical Research Council and the World Health Organization, suggests that children should not have dental X-rays without good reason, as their thyroid glands are especially sensitive to radiation.

Nurseries, schools, colleges and leisure centres

Our recommendations

🗑 Rooms with **low ceilings and fluorescent lights** may have readings above 0.2 microtesla at head height. In multistorey schools with fluorescent lights, young children may be far enough away from the ceiling fixtures, but may still be exposed to EMFs from the lights installed in rooms below.

For information on computers, including wLAN systems, laboratories and interactive whiteboards, see Chapters 4, 5 and 7.

?? Many leisure facilities, such as **cinemas, multiplexes, bowling alleys, discos, clubs** and the like, can have a great deal of ambient EMFs. While this may not be a problem for most people, those with EHS are likely to be badly affected.

Exposure to EMFs when travelling and out and about in the community can be very variable. The information in this chapter is intended to help you become aware of some of the sources you are commonly likely to encounter, what you can do about them, and how you can make more informed choices.

We can not cover every eventuality, but you will have a better idea of the sort of things to look out for and the questions to ask.

Reducing levels when out and about

DO

✔ Make sure you do not stay for long in a place with high radiofrequency radiation. Check with a monitor if you are unsure of the levels.

✔ Try to limit your shopping to places where they do not have all the latest stock control gadgetry. Check field levels if you are unsure.

✔ Think carefully about what medical procedures you choose to have, including ultrasound scans, especially if these are for 'routine' purposes only.

✔ Hold out for an MRI scan rather than a CAT scan, if possible.

✔ Be cautious about diathermy treatment.

✔ If you need to go to hospital, think about whether you wish to expose yourself to EMFs from the Patientline equipment. Try to keep it at least 50 centimetres away when watching it.

DON'T

✗ Don't stand near security pillars in shops or elsewhere.

✗ Do not use internet and broadband cafes if you have EHS.

✗ Don't have routine dental X-rays and refuse them for your children unless there is a pressing diagnostic reason.

7

Pregnancy, Children and EMFs

If you're thinking of starting a family or are already a parent, this chapter is for you.

You'll have noted that in many of our recommendations, the general rule is that pregnant women and children are far more vulnerable to EMFs, and need to take extra care – or avoid certain places altogether. In this chapter, we'll look in more detail at the issues parents, parents-to-be and people thinking about having a child will need to consider in relation to EMFs.

For men, sperm damage and partial sterility could be a concern. For women – particularly at the time of conception and in the first trimester of pregnancy – the health risks are much more wide-ranging and complex. And once your child is born, there are new EMF hazards.

Much of the experimentation into EMFs and health has been carried out in laboratories using specially cultured cells or animals. It is not certain whether the results of this research reflect what really happens to people. Epidemiological studies, which are surveys of health in real populations, have not usually focused on specific exposures experienced by pregnant women. We have to make educated guesses much of the time that take into account the particular vulnerabilities of young, actively growing bodies.

Conception to birth

Many of us learned about 'simple' genetics at school and remember that genes are passed on from parents to their children, that people carry dominant and recessive genes, and that everything is recorded in, and controlled by, DNA. But the study of genetics has moved on, and in truth, it's all a lot more complex than this.

Inherited DNA carries not only direct information – so if you have gene A from both parents you will have blue eyes, and if you have gene B from one or both you will have brown ones. It also carries 'switches' that control whether this information is actually used in the development of the body. These can be turned on or off by illnesses or the parents' exposure to substances or forces in the environment. This discovery is recent and the importance of it in human development has only just been recognised.

This new area of genetics is called epigenetics. Many scientists now believe that 'incorrect' epigenetic changes are some of the first steps in cancer initiation. One gene changed in this way, that can be passed on from a parent, can result in retinoblastoma and leukaemia developing in children. As we've seen, the incidence of childhood leukaemia is associated with EMF exposure.

More and more is being found out about the complex interaction of genes since we started mapping the human genome. And as our knowledge grows, it is going to prove far more complicated still. (For more information on epigenetics, see the Appendix.)

In the context of EMFs and human health, one of the implications of epigenetics is very significant. It is often said that the kind of non-ionising radiation we look at in this book does not have the energy to damage DNA. If such EMFs affect genetic switches in people, changing the way their genes work, these changes can also be passed on to any children they may have.

This means that you should be very careful of your exposure to EMFs and other stresses if you are thinking of trying for a baby. It's best to begin right when you start trying to conceive, as it can be some weeks before a woman is aware she's pregnant – and that is the most vulnerable time for the foetus. The effects of EMFs, chemicals and viruses seem to be strongest during the first trimester of pregnancy, whereas stress hormones, such as cortisol, play a far more active role in the third trimester.

Problems with fertility

Low sperm counts and problems with conception in general have been much in the news for some years now. But how much are EMFs to blame in this growing problem?

In 1985, a study found that 1 in 6 married couples had fertility problems and the numbers were increasing. In a 1989 study, 25 per cent of women under 30, and 40 per cent over 30, were found to be mainly infertile. Men are not exempt from the problem as the sperm count of men studied in America has fallen by more than 30 per cent over the last 50 years. Some 25 per cent of men now have sperm counts so low that they are functionally sterile.

Many people believe that it is likely to be environmental pollutants that are having this effect. The joint WWF and
Greenpeace report *A Present for Life: Hazardous chemicals in
cord blood*, published in September 2005, highlights the fact
that our babies are being exposed to a huge range of chemicals at the most vulnerable point in their development. Every
single sample of the 40 mother's and 35 baby's blood tested
positive for an array of chemicals, many of which are
suspected of links to health problems ranging from birth
defects and genital abnormalities to certain types of cancer.
Most of the chemicals are found in products that we all use
every day, like cleaning fluids and sprays, tin can linings,
perfumes, cosmetics and even baby bottles.

But chemical pollutants don't necessarily act in isolation, and
the most likely culprit behind the level of infertility we are
seeing is probably a synergistic mix of the chemicals with
EMFs and other factors, such as lifestyle. Certainly, since 1977
studies have shown that EMFs at powerfrequency and radiofrequency are affecting sperm quality and motility. The
scientific literature over the last 20 years is increasingly
showing that chromosomal abnormalities, abnormal foetal
development and genetic conditions such as Down syndrome
are found to be more common among people exposed to
EMFs either in their workplace or home.

If you are planning on starting a family, and especially if you
have been trying for some time with no luck, it is worth
checking your use of electrical and radiofrequency appliances
in the home and to minimise exposure wherever possible in
the workplace. A good source of relevant information is
Foresight (see Resources).

r■ ■ ■ ■ ■ ■ ■ ■ ■ ■ ■ ■ ■ ■ ■ ■ ■ ■

Preparing for pregnancy

When preparing for pregnancy we suggest that you
reduce your exposure to EMFs, including the following:

✔ Check your house for electrical appliances that
   may be too near sitting/sleeping places, before
   you start trying to conceive.
✔ Check your work exposure to EMFs and
   minimise if possible.
✔ Keep mobile phone and laptop computer use to
   a minimum when planning a pregnancy.
✔ Choose and use environmentally friendly cleaning
   products and locally produced organic foods whenever you can. Less and best is the way to go.

Problems in pregnancy

Most pregnancies are still successful, but miscarriage is far
more common than many people realise. In 1988, the US
National Institute of Environmental Health Sciences (NIEHS)
found that 31 per cent of pregnancies ended in miscarriage.
They suspected that some unknown form of environmental
pollution or stress was the cause.

Two epidemiology studies published in 2000 and 2002 suggest
that a substantial proportion of miscarriages (40 per cent)
might be caused by maternal EMF exposure. They theorised
that the added risk of miscarriage for a pregnant woman
exposed to EMFs may be 5 to 10 per cent.

Overall, Dr De-Kun Li and his team for the 2002 study found
that women exposed to peak levels of 1.6 microtesla or greater

were nearly twice as likely to miscarry as women not exposed to such strong fields.[38] More significantly, among the 622 women who said the measuring period had been 'a typical day', those who experienced EMFs with occasional very high levels such as those from electric trains and motorised home appliances, were three times as likely to have a miscarriage. 'That's another confirmation that the effect is due to EMF,' said Li. Exposure to more than 1.6 microtesla in the first 10 weeks of pregnancy increased the risk of miscarriage by 6 times.

Li's study showed a strong link between vacuum cleaner usage and increased risk of miscarriage. The finding prompted Li to caution pregnant women to 'at least do a cost-benefit analysis if using a vacuum cleaner is part of your profession. If it's just at home, I would consider not using a vacuum cleaner because there are certain things that can be done to avoid it – other people can do it.'

In late 2005, Dr Li received a grant from the NIEHS to continue his work. Surprisingly, no funding has been made available in Europe to pay for similar studies.

There have been many laboratory and animal studies looking at the effects of low-frequency and high-frequency EMFs on egg and foetal development. These have found many more congenital abnormalities, stillbirths and spontaneous abortions in high exposure conditions. In one, nine pregnant squirrels and monkeys were exposed to EMFs at or below the US safety standard, while nine were kept free of exposure. Five of the exposed young died within six months, while there were no deaths among the young of the group not exposed to EMFs.

Maureen Asbury and the Trentham Environmental Action Campaign (UK, Stoke on Trent, see Resources) have carried out two studies on health near overhead powerlines and found greatly increased miscarriage rates in women living within 150 metres of the lines.

We feel that overall, while the links are not conclusively proven, due care regarding EMFs is needed when you're pregnant. Let's look at how, now.

Care in pregnancy

As we've seen, it's the first trimester of pregnancy that is the key period for reducing any environmental risks. If you're pregnant, it is vital to take the sort of precautions discussed in Chapter 4 regarding all electrical appliances throughout the house, and to identify and avoid sources of high EMFs.

Our recommendations

In the home
🗑 Keep away from all equipment while it is working, especially those at the same height as your 'bump', as the growing foetus could be directly affected, and at your head height, where EMFs could affect your immune system and your health.

Reducing your exposure during pregnancy

DO

✔ Keep at least 1 metre from the front of televisions. The side and back give off higher EMFs. Put the TV in a position where there is no (or no easy) access to the rear and side.
✔ Keep a reasonable distance from computers – do not use a laptop actually on your lap.

✔ Minimise your use of electric appliances at worktop height in the kitchen.

✔ Move clock radios at least 1 metre away from your pillow.

✔ Be cautious about continuing to follow an occupation where high exposure levels from electrical or electronic equipment is the norm – such as physiotherapy, welding or industrial sewing.

✔ Reduce your use of electric household appliances such as vacuum cleaners, food mixers or other motorised equipment that you need to stand close to.

✔ Check your car for high EMFs. Some models, especially those with the batteries in the boot/trunk away from the engine, are particularly problematic.

✔ If you have powerlines over, or a substation next to, your garden, avoid sitting in their vicinity.

✔ Keep storage radiators away from beds, including beds behind walls.

DON'T

✗ Don't hold a cordless phone or mobile phone near to your 'bump'. Preferably do not use one at all, for your own benefit.

✗ Don't wear support bras that contain metal. These can act as passive antennas near radiofrequency sources such as mobile phones, and can microwave your breasts.

✗ Avoid standing near a working microwave oven, or close to the front of an electric cooker or washing machine when in use.

✗ Don't use a hairdryer in the evening: it is likely to have an effect on the immune system and

your body's damage repair mechanisms. Do not hold it next to the growing foetus at any time.
- ✗ **Never leave any type of electric blanket turned on when you've got into bed.**
- ✗ **Try not to travel on electric trains more than you have to, especially in the first three months of pregnancy.**

Out and about

Outside sources of EMFs should be carefully avoided where possible. Chapter 2 discusses the risks from powerlines, cables, substations, mobile phone masts and their equipment cabins and so on, while in Chapter 6 you'll find information about the different places where you may encounter high levels of EMFs when travelling and out and about generally.

As we've seen, it is abrupt changes in magnetic fields that are of specific concern to pregnant women when travelling in electric trains, as these shifts are associated with an increased risk of miscarriage in the first and possibly the second trimester.

?? There are places with very high EMFs in trains – see Chapter 6. As trains vary so much in design and construction, the only way to find these places is to carry a small EMF monitor with you at all times (available from EMFields, see Resources).

?? Cars can have both high levels of EMFs and high microwave levels, as we saw in Chapter 6. As a general rule, the older and cheaper the model of car, the better it is in terms of EMFs. There can be high EMFs above the wheel arches in cars and buses because wheels and tyres are frequently unintentionally magnetised during manufacture.

Care of newborns and young babies

Although the high-tech monitoring and heating devices in hospital nurseries routinely expose many newborns to high EMFs, it is important to remember the advantages here – and the consequences to your baby's health if this level of care wasn't given.

This doesn't mean we can ignore the results of some studies. One has found that children with SIDS (sudden infant death syndrome) had lower levels of melatonin, the hormone produced at night by the pineal gland. Melatonin is extremely sensitive to EMFs. And a hospital in San Diego, California, found that 14 out of 18 autistic children had lesions in the brain identical to those in rats exposed to EMFs between one and six days after birth.

So reasonable care needs to be taken, and here we examine the things worth looking out for.

Our recommendations

In the kitchen

🗑 🗑 🗑 ☺ ☺

If you are bottlefeeding your baby, do not use an **electric bottle warmer** unless it has a three-core cable (which means it is earthed). Unearthed bottle warmers can give off high electric fields.

🗑 🗑 🗑 🗑 🗑

Do not heat stored breast milk, formula or any other baby food in a **microwave oven**. Microwaving milk releases the rogue molecules known as free radicals and may create toxic chemicals, associated with cancers, and also alters amino acid and protein structures. The effects of this are uncertain, but it is

wise to avoid creating this problem, as amino acids are used
as building materials in your child's body.

In the bedroom
The two primary EMF concerns in the bedroom are baby
monitors, and nightlights – which carry an added risk. There is
plenty of strong scientific evidence that shows that even quite
low levels of light stop the production of melatonin, a hormonal
chemical synthesised in the pineal gland. It, and its associated
chemicals, 'mop up' dangerous free-radical damage. There is
good evidence that low levels of melatonin increase the likelihood of cancers and other serious health problems developing.

It is often your anxiety about seeing your child that starts the
'light at night' habit. Remember that your child will have been in
virtual darkness until they were born. It is all too easy for you to
unintentionally condition them to wanting a light on at night. The
only type of nightlight that you should use are the very low power
(usually plug mounted) orange or red ones that just glow gently.
Red and orange lights hardly affect the production of melatonin,
but white and blue-white lights are likely to stop the pineal
gland's production of melatonin for the whole of the night.

☺ ☺ ☺ ☺ ☺
Battery-operated, wire-connected baby monitors give off virtually
zero EMFs and are the best in this context.

🗑 🗑 ☺ ☺ ☺
Baby monitors that are **plugged into the mains** can give off
significant amounts of EMF radiation. They should be at least
1 metre away from the baby's head.

🗑 🗑 🗑 🗑 ☺
The **'walkabout' wireless 'freedom' alarms** give off high levels of
radiofrequency radiation next to the child to communicate with

the parents' listening unit. These should be used with great caution, if at all. Some, though, have very low fields. We recommend that before buying one, you test it in the shop using a microwave radiation monitor that can check for power level and digital pulsing. Some analogue units are probably fine, but avoid DECT units (see page 83).

> We had the following communication from a father who was horrified to discover the levels of microwaves his and his sister's babies had been sleeping in.
>
> Since she was born, our daughter has had a digital DECT baby monitor in her room. She has suffered from very restless sleep, often crying out but not waking, or waking and crying, and also twisting herself about in her cot until she gets trapped in the corners which again wakes her up. I used the Powerwatch designed COM monitor and found readings in the red – 4V/m – in her cot. We bought an analogue monitor to replace the DECT digital one and since then she has slept very peacefully every night. I told my sister, who was also experiencing the same problems; she also replaced her monitor with an analogue one and now her son sleeps like a log. This is surely not coincidence.

Sensor pads, which are put under the mattress with the intention of monitoring the baby's breathing, etc, should be used with great care. One well-known UK make was found to produce significant levels of pulsing microwaves around the baby's body. If you wish to use this form of monitoring, which can help to prevent sudden infant death syndrome, we strongly recommend that you check them even more stringently for microwaves than the normal walkabout monitors. You should also check them for powerfrequency electric fields.

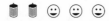

Make sure that wherever your baby sleeps, he or she is at least 1 metre from the nearest electrical appliance (including music players).

Dimmer switches can give off significant electric fields and radiofrequency noise, so if you feel you need to use one of these, it should be kept well away from the baby's head. It would be best to switch a dim orange or red light on when you want dim lighting.

If you decide you really do need to have a light on in your child's bedroom overnight, a plug-based, extremely low-power, glowing orange nightlight is best.

In the garden

In the UK, there's a time-honoured tradition of putting babies out in a pram in the garden for a daytime nap. Fresh air is indeed healthful, but if your property is next to a substation or its underground cables, or there are powerlines across your garden or near the garden, make sure your baby sleeps as far away from them as possible.

If there is a source of high-frequency radiation (a mobile phone mast, a cordless phone in a neighbour's house, an amateur radio operator or the like), check the garden for areas of low exposure and ensure the baby sleeps in one of these, or screen the pram using special RF protective netting (see Resources, EMFields).

Reducing exposure for young babies

DO

✔ Use a battery-operated, wire-connected baby monitor.

✔ Keep a plug-in alarm at least 1 metre away from the baby's head.

✔ If you intend to use a 'walkabout' alarm, use care when selecting it.

✔ Encourage your baby to sleep in a darkened room.

✔ If you feel there must be a light in the baby's bedroom, use a plug-based, extremely low-power orange glowing nightlight.

✔ Arrange your baby's sleeping area so that he or she is at least a metre from the nearest electric appliance.

✔ Check your garden for areas with the lowest EMF levels as sites for your baby's pram.

DON'T

✘ Avoid using an electric bottle warmer to heat breast milk or formula.

✘ Don't heat formula or any other baby food in a microwave oven.

✘ Don't use a digital cordless monitor, unless you have measured the fields and found them to be low. These can give off high levels of microwaves, which affect some babies significantly.

✘ Avoid using a sensor pad under the cot mattress

unless you have measured the microwave emissions and found them to be low.

✗ Don't use a dimmer switch to provide a light in the baby's sleeping room, unless it is well away from the baby's head. Ensure the bulb it is lighting is red or orange, not white or bluish.

Care of growing children

Helping your child avoid EMF exposure as he or she grows is important, but it is not the whole story when it comes to health. By paying attention to a range of factors, from TV use to diet, you can boost your child's growth and vitality to optimal levels.

For instance, Roberto Salti and colleagues at the University of Florence in Italy found that when 74 children aged 6 to 12 were deprived of their TVs and computers for a week and other sources of artificial light were reduced in their homes, their production of melatonin (see text above) increased by an average of 30 per cent. The increases were highest in the youngest children.

And, according to a recent MORI survey, 1 in 20 children aged 11 to 16 claim to have eaten no vegetables, and 1 in 17 no fruit, in the previous week. Most of the children claimed to have eaten fewer than 13 portions of fruit or vegetables. Most authorities now recommend five portions a day to help prevent obesity, cancer and heart disease.

Our recommendations

In the kitchen and living room

We do not believe that **microwave ovens** (see Chapter 4) should be used to cook your child's food or warm their drinks, except on very rare occasions. If you do use a microwave, ensure the food or drink is taken out when it is too hot. This way, it has to be left outside the oven for a minimum of two minutes for it to be cool enough to consume, which will allow any free radicals to disappear.

When using electrical appliances such as **cookers, washing machines, tumble dryers, dishwashers** and so on, which can give off high levels of EMFs, do not let your child play in front of them.

Make your child sit at least a metre from the **TV** (see Chapter 4). As well as the EMFs TVs can give off, TV screens also carry electrostatic fields, which can attract dust including chemical particles, bacteria, viruses and the like.

If your child wants to use a **computer**, ensure they sit at a comfortable arm's length. Young children should not spend much time on it. The use of computers generates positive ions, and generally we feel much better in an atmosphere rich in negative ions; excessive computer use may be able to initiate electrical hypersensitivity, a highly debilitating condition.

Do not let young children have a toy **mobile phone**. It's best if your child never associates them with 'fun'. Research is increasingly showing that using mobile phones is hazardous and can lead to serious illnesses, as well as behavioural distur-bances and concentration and memory problems.

Do not let your child use a **digital cordless phone**, which carries the same risks as a mobile phone as it uses the same technology.

🗑 🗑 🗑 ☺ ☺

Many electrically powered toys come with a **transformer**, a small black box you plug into a socket. These can give off very high fields, so do not plug them in next to a bed.

🗑 🗑 ☺ ☺ ☺

Batteries used in many toys and other equipment do not give off high EMFs. However, they can contain mercury, cadmium, lithium and other toxic, non-biodegradable metals that can affect water supplies from landfill, potentially poisoning your child's environment. Long-term, low-level exposure to cadmium residues in air, water and food can cause kidney disease, lung damage and brittle bones. They are not energy-efficient: manufacturing them uses 50 times more energy than they will ever produce. Re-chargeable batteries should be used and then recycled if possible. It is better to consider your overall use of power-driven appliances, than just to replace mains-operated equipment with battery-operated ones.

In the bedroom
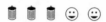

One study has shown that children who used **electric blankets** were more likely to develop leukaemia, the commonest form of childhood cancer. Using an electric blanket to warm the bed, and unplugging it when your child gets in, might work, but having an electric blanket on the bed could tempt a child to switch it on while they were in the bed – and as we've seen, this is not advisable (see page 105).

Do not put your child's bedhead next to the **immersion heater** or the **meter cupboard**. High fields come from the equipment including the wiring. In **blocks of flats**, make sure the bed is not close to the main services riser – the place where the cables and pipes run vertically up through the building.

Make sure **bedside lights and wires** are kept away from the pillow area. If your child sleeps on the top bunk bed, make sure there is no **dimmer switch** near the pillow.

There are frequently high electric fields from wiring. If your child's bedroom is on an upper floor, the wiring to the lights in the room below will lead to your child being in high fields when they play on the floor. You can reduce the fields using earthed aluminium foil on the floor underneath any floor covering.

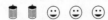

Music centres and mains CD players can give off high EMFs. Ensure the system has a decent electrical earth connection to the mains supply and keep a metre away when listening to them.

Personal radios and stereos, including MP3 players, do not pose an EMF problem when run on batteries. Headphones attached by a lead to musical equipment are fine as long as the equipment itself is earthed. If it is unearthed, the head-phones will give off high electric fields.

Remote cordless headphone systems have a microwave trans-mitter attached to the base unit. The receiver is in the headset worn by the person listening. Headsets are safe, but the transmitter gives off microwave fields. Sit a reasonable distance away from the transmitting unit.

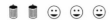

If your child has a **lamp** on a table next to her or him a lot while occupied with hobbies, ensure that the lamp is earthed. Most table lamps aren't and can give off quite high electric fields.

☺ ☺ ☺ ☺ ☺

Most electrically powered **exercise equipment** has the motor near less vulnerable parts of the body, although pregnant women shouldn't use motor-driven walking exercisers. They are not a problem for general use, though exercising outside is usually a better option in any case.

In the garden

If your child spends a lot of time in the garden playing, reading, sleeping and so on, look out for sources of EMFs, especially **powerlines, substations, underground cables and mobile phone masts**. If your garden is close to any of these, we recommend that you measure the EMFs and find areas in the garden with low readings. Encourage your children to play there, or make them into special play areas.

Out in the community

?? When with your child on **public transport** (trains, trams or buses), do not let them sit in the seats directly above the wheel arches (see Chapter 6).

🗑 Do not carry a mobile phone on standby in a bag hanging on a child's **pushchair**.

🗑 The **security devices** in shops and libraries give off very high EMFs at child height. Do not let your child play inside the security walkways or near them, and do not leave a pushchair next to them.

🗑 The thyroid glands of children are especially sensitive to radiation. Children should not have **dental X-rays** without good reason (see Chapter 1).

Schools and nurseries

?? Electromagnetic fields in nurseries and schools can be highly variable. Large buildings may have their own substations that cause local areas of high EMFs nearby. Care should be taken to ensure that areas regularly used by children should have low ambient EMFs. Occasionally nurseries provided in the workplace for the convenience of employees may be situated on floors above basement substations. These will create very high levels of EMFs to the side and on floors immediately above.

?? Many schools and nurseries use fluorescent lighting, which as we've seen can generate EMFs and, occasionally, significant levels of RF radiation. The flicker can trigger electrical hyper-sensitivity and increase antisocial behaviour.

If your child develops headaches and/or eye strain, check the school classroom lighting. It is important, if at all possible, to ensure that the lights are full-spectrum lights, as it has been found that people are much healthier and thus able to learn better in lighting that approximates daylight as closely as possible.

Where children's daily programme includes a time for a rest or sleep, we recommend that the illumination in the room should be kept as low as possible, as this ensures better quality of rest.

🗑 🗑 🗑 🗑 🗑

Toy mobile phones have no place in nurseries or schools, as they can predispose children to wanting to own the real thing. Many countries prohibit the sale of mobile phones to children, and the UK Department of Health recommends that children under 16 should only use mobile phones in an emergency. Research from Scandinavia has shown that brain cells can be damaged beyond repair by mobile phone radiation, resulting in a form of dementia.[39]

?? Acquiring high-tech equipment has become a major goal for many schools, as they feel this is a way of offering better opportunities to their students. It can be – but the risks do need to be weighed up.

Although modern computer monitors emit low EMFs, the time children spend playing on computers should be restricted. Usage is linked to eye strain, repetitive strain injury (RSI), and electrical hypersensitivity. While computers constitute a valuable tool and it is obviously important to learn to use them, they should be treated with caution from the beginning.

?? Some primary schools are beginning to encourage the use of laptops among their pupils as a convenient way of researching topics on the internet. As mentioned previously, however, laptops can give off high fields if not earthed. The way the screens display the pictures has changed, and although the images look better, they may now be just as likely to create eye strain problems as they used to be.

🗑 In some classrooms, computers are networked via a wireless local area network (wLAN) system, where a central control mechanism uses pulsing microwaves to communicate with the computers. We are very concerned about children being exposed to such high microwave fields.

☺ We recommend that computer networks are connected with cables. Find out what kind of network, if any, your child's school uses, and if it is wireless, campaign for a safer system.

?? Interactive whiteboards in the classroom can increase children's exposure to microwave radiation. The projector is not a problem but the portable sketch pads, which can be moved from table to table for the children to draw and write on, communicate using pulsing microwave technology.

As microwave exposure is associated with memory and concentration problems as well as behaviour and mood disturbances, we believe further research should be done before the widespread use of these systems in our places of learning is encouraged. Perhaps some investigation by the school or PTA would be useful in quantifying the effect, if any. Changes in children's performance or behaviour could be monitored.

Reducing your child's exposure

DO

✔ Minimise the time your children play computer games.

✔ Monitor the type of games they play.

✔ Keep children at least a metre away from working electrical appliances in the kitchen.

✔ Make sure your child sits at least a metre away from the front of a TV screen while watching.

✔ Position the television set so children cannot spend time to the side or back of it.

✔ Make sure transformers are kept away from chairs, beds and anywhere a child sits and plays regularly.

✔ Consider your use of battery-operated equipment. Use rechargeable batteries where possible and dispose of them as toxic waste.

✔ Position your child's bed away from cupboards containing electric equipment, meters, heaters and the like.

✔ Make sure all music players are earthed.

✔ Make sure your child sits well away from the transmitting unit of a cordless headphone system.

✔ Make sure desk and bedside table lamps are earthed.

✔ Check your garden for EMF sources and build play areas where field levels are low.

✔ Make sure your child sits in seats that are not exposed to high EMFs in public transport.

✔ Check your child's nursery and school for sources of EMFs.

✔ Monitor your child's health, behaviour and achievement levels and check school EMF exposure if these deteriorate.

✔ Check whether your child's school has a wireless LAN system or interactive whiteboards. Measure the EMFs in the classroom to see if they are at an acceptable level.

DON'T

✘ Don't use a microwave oven to cook food or heat drinks.

✘ Don't encourage your child to play with a toy mobile phone.

✘ Don't let your child talk on a digital cordless (DECT) phone.

✘ Avoid warming your child's bed with an electric blanket.

✗ Keep wires and lights away from your child's pillow area and don't keep anything electric – especially mains-powered tape players – near the head of your child's bed.

✗ Don't allow your child to play on the floor of an upstairs room without checking EMF levels first.

✗ Don't build a play area or tree house in an area of the garden which could be exposed to high EMF levels.

✗ Don't carry a mobile phone on standby on the handle of a pushchair near your child's head.

✗ Keep your child from playing near security walkway passages in shops, libraries and the like.

8

What to Do if You're Electrosensitive

Imagine feeling pain or nausea every time you came within a few feet of a mobile phone or computer, or when you entered a car or train. Given that our 21st-century world is literally crammed with appliances, equipment and vehicles that emit EMFs, such a scenario is almost unimaginable – one long, fraught obstacle course. Yet it's a daily reality for people with electrical hypersensitivity, or EHS.

EHS is not yet a widely recognised condition, and it is often dismissed as psychosomatic or labelled as a psychiatric problem. We feel it is important to give sufferers a voice. Here are some of their stories.

Gro Harlem Brundtland, who has served as Norway's prime minister and director-general of the World Health Organization (WHO), and is also a medical doctor, suffers from EHS. She gets headaches every time she's near a mobile phone, and has become so sensitive to mobile phone radiation that people within 4 metres of her must turn their phones off in order to stop her from feeling ill. She thought she could avoid the pain by reducing the time she spent on her mobile, but this hasn't helped. In 2004, when she told the world of her EHS, she was fortunate that the headaches she was getting as a result of the radiation went away within half an hour to an hour after the EMF source was moved away or turned off.

Brundtland also reacts to her laptop PC. If she holds it to read the screen, she says, 'It feels like I get an electric shock through my arms.' She adds, 'We do not know whether this sensitivity can lead to serious outcomes such as cancer or other diseases, but I am convinced this must be taken seriously.'

Ian, in charge of a highly successful company in the UK food industry with a turnover of hundreds of millions of pounds per year, is another sufferer.

I have become highly electrosensitive, to the extent that I have had to remove all electronic equipment from my office and use a 1950s telephone. When I have business meetings, I have to ask the other people to turn off their mobile phones.

When I look back, I had used a mobile phone regularly for about 15 years. First analogue, and then various digital ones. It was in 1999 that I first realised that I wasn't feeling so well if I had been on the phone for more than a few minutes, but didn't really take it on board. By the end of the year I was regularly getting strange sensations and had reduced my mobile phone use. Some time towards the end of 2000 I got severe pain during one particular call followed by a blinding headache. Since then I have been electrosensitive. I have had brain scans and there doesn't seem to be anything physically wrong that can be seen.

I didn't know there was such a thing as electrosensitivity. I just knew that I got severe pain when anybody near me used a mobile phone. I then started to get the same sort of sensations around electrical equipment. It was some time later that my wife went onto the internet and pulled off details about electrosensitivity, and we ticked off many of the reported symptoms. At last I was able to put a name to what it appeared I had and I learnt that it was recognised by some people.

If I keep away from electromagnetic fields then I am completely OK. Keeping away from electrical equipment in today's society is almost impossible. If I become highly exposed, on a trip to London for example, then I will be very poorly for at least 24 hours afterwards, so I have to plan my work life very carefully. I struggle to use a computer and so rarely do, don't watch TV, cinema, travel on electric trains, or air flights with in-seat entertainment – cheap charter flights are generally OK, interestingly enough.

I can't use a modern car – I have tried many, from the cheapest to top luxury models, which are often the worst! I can't visit other people's homes if they have a cordless telephone. There are certain areas in the back of our house towards the distant mast (over half a mile away) which I cannot go into. I take holidays in the UK in areas well out of the way of masts – I have to check for pylons and masts in the area before we go. We rent detached properties where we can turn off the electricity when we don't need to use it.

There is very little awareness about electrosensitivity. What you find if you go to your doctor will be that he is likely to say that such a condition does not exist, that the effects you are reporting must be psychosomatic. So electrosensitive people generally go to ground and use alternative therapists because the mainstream medical profession refuses to recognise that this can happen. This situation will have to change as more and more people seem to be reporting symptoms of electrosensitivity.

Margaret used to be a secondary school teacher. She began to feel quite poorly when using her computer, though she did not know why. Then she also began to feel ill walking down the school corridors. She was off sick for a few days, but returned to work when she started to feel better. Immediately she began to feel ill again. Her work colleagues put it down to stress at work and were sympathetic, up to a point. Margaret was sure it was not stress but something else. She then developed thyroid problems.

Searching the internet, she became convinced her symptoms pointed to EHS, as she felt better when away from sources of electromagnetic radiation such as computers and fluorescent lights. She contacted Powerwatch and a thyroid self-help group, and began to piece together the jigsaw of her experiences. The education authorities did not accept her self-diagnosis of EHS, her GP was unsympathetic, her union did not feel she had a case, and she had to take early retirement on the grounds of ill health. She has since become an active campaigner for the recognition of EHS.

Anatomy of EHS

EHS can affect anyone, and some quite badly. The symptoms are listed in the questionnaire in Chapter 1, and you may recognise that you develop some of them – numbness, prickling or pain, for instance – when you're near sources of EMFs.

If you have EHS, some of the symptoms will noticeably appear or get worse near electrical appliances, powerlines, underground cables, fluorescent or halogen lights, mobile phones, digital cordless phones, mobile phone base stations and/or other electromagnetic field sources, and diminish (or occasionally disappear) away from the source of EMFs.

EHS can vary from individual to individual. The severity of your symptoms may be different from that of other sufferers. You might find that you feel worse in some places, such as at work, and not in others. Stress-sensitive hormones such as prolactin and thyroxine are higher in people who work in electromagnetic environments and in EHS sufferers when they are near the EMF sources they're sensitive to.

It may take some time for the symptoms to disappear after you reduce your exposure. With mild cases of EHS, this may happen in a few days. It was suggested at a 2003 seminar on EHS held at the Royal College of Medicine in London that three months may have to be allowed between an acute response to an EMF source and re-exposure to it.

Nobody knows as yet whether EHS is a separate condition, or just one in a constellation of general environmental sensitivity syndromes which includes multiple chemical sensitivity (MCS), sick-building syndrome (SBS), asthma, fibromyalgia, chronic fatigue syndrome (CFS) and myalgic encephalomyelitis (ME, a sub-set of CFS). There is some evidence that ME can be triggered by electric fields.

If you suffer from EHS, the chances are that you also react to chemicals and/or have intolerance to some types of food, such as gluten or dairy products.

As long ago as 1990, Dr Robert Becker, a pioneer in the field of EMFs and health effects, showed in his book *Cross Currents* that there are neurological similarities between symptoms of chronic fatigue syndrome, multiple chemical sensitivity syndrome (MCS) and EHS. These symptoms show that the body's systems for dealing with stress are breaking down. When EHS sufferers live in a high EMF environment, it is like a person with auditory sensitivity trying to carry on normal life with someone shouting in both ears all the time.

Who is vulnerable?

Kjell Hansson Mild of the National Institute for Working Life in Sweden, one of the foremost researchers into EHS, believes that there is a particular group of people who are sensitive to environmental influences, and that if you are in that group, you are likely to develop more than one adverse reaction. You may have various food allergies, you may suffer from asthma or hay fever. Mild thinks that the majority, though not all, of EHS people could fall into this group.

Dr Hajime Kimata from Unitika Hospital in Kyoto, Japan, believes microwaves emitted by mobile phone handsets can 'excite' antigens – the substances that trigger allergic reactions – in the bloodstream of people who already suffer from allergies.

Interestingly in the light of this theory, mast cells – which play a large role in various types of well-known allergic reactions, such as asthma – have been seen to increase in the skin of healthy volunteers sitting in front of some computer monitors. We do not know if it is the EMFs from the screen or the unusual quality of the light that is responsible. Modern cathode ray tube monitors (ie not flat screen TFT ones) that have crisp stable displays are actually flashing very brightly at a rate that is too fast to be seen.

Olle Johansson of the Karolinska Institute in Stockholm, Sweden, has investigated numbers of people suffering from exposure to computer monitors (VDUs) and other EMF sources.[40] Many of these people first suffer from skin irritation such as itching, heat sensations and reddening. In some of these people Johansson has clear evidence showing peripheral damage in the nerve endings found within 0.010 to 0.020 millimetres of the skin surface. The normal purpose of these nerve fibres is unclear, but it does appear they are involved in at least some cases of EHS.

The nerve endings seem to become super-sensitive and react both more quickly and more intensely to external stimuli, especially electric fields and some chemicals. It is known that new electronic equipment, including computers, give off significant levels of volatile organic fire-retardant chemicals that can mimic natural body messenger chemicals, and these are believed to be involved in the triggering of EHS in some people.

In Sweden, there is a phenomenal increase in asthma among youngsters up to 18 years of age. It is thought this may be the result of an allergic reaction to the extensive use of computer equipment. The finding we have mentioned elsewhere in this book, about static fields generated by computer monitors attracting pollutants such as bacteria and viruses, may make this kind of reaction worse.

There is some evidence that having metallic dental fillings, caps and so on – such as gold or stainless steel crowns, mercury amalgam and titanium crown posts – may be a significant factor in many older people's EHS. Metallic mixtures can cause electro-chemical potentials to be set up in the mouth to which some people react.

Chemical exposure is a major cause of fatigue, depression and poor concentration. R.A. Buist, author of the book *Chronic Fatigue Syndrome and Chemical Overload*, points out that toxins can disrupt the way muscles work, which may account for the pain and weakness of muscles experienced by many people who suffer from EHS.

EHS can be triggered by just one instance of exposure, such as a call on a new mobile phone; or by a series of exposures, such as working at a particular computer monitor for a number of weeks.

British biophysicist Peter Alexander has said, 'Once the individual is sensitised to an agent, the initial aggressor is immaterial. The biological reaction will be the same to all agents.'

Bill Curry, a US-based EMF physicist and bio-effects expert, believes that anyone subjected to microwave radiation on a regular basis will eventually become electrosensitive.

Living with EHS: a look at the triggers

For people with EHS, daily life can become extremely difficult, and a 'normal' existence virtually impossible in severe cases. Fluorescent lights, for instance, are used in public offices, shops, libraries, theatres, cinemas, internet cafés, concert halls, restau- rants, churches, meeting rooms, doctors' and dentists' surgeries, trains, planes, trams and buses (see also Chapters 5 and 6). Neighbours with digital cordless phones or who are amateur radio operators can unwittingly make an EHS neighbour's life almost unbearable. A nearby mobile phone mast can make a house uninhabitable. If you suffer from EHS you may not even be able to go down a road where one of these masts is situated.

Children are increasingly exposed to computers and fluores- cent lights at an early age, even in pre-school nurseries. We are very concerned that a number will develop this sensitivity with all the restrictions that go along with it.

People with EHS can react to EMFs from a huge range of sources:

- Televisions
- Mobile and digital cordless phones
- Fluorescent lights
- Computer monitors (VDTs, VDUs)
- Laptop computers, when used with mains adapters
- Powerlines

- Substations
- Mobile phone base station masts
- Underground electric cables
- Electric fields due to house wiring
- Telephones, answering machines and faxes
- Some new, upmarket cars, especially those equipped with RF CANBUS, or Bluetooth-enabled systems
- Electrical 'noise' in trains, underground trains, trams, buses and cars
- Wireless enabled laptops
- Electronic 'anti-theft' tagging scanners at the exits to many department stores.
- Refrigerators
- Freezers
- Electric cookers (including induction hobs)
- Vacuum cleaners
- Battery-operated appliances
- Fish tank heaters or lights
- Photocopiers
- Lamps with attached or built-in transformers
- Dimmer switches
- Burglar alarms
- Low-energy, mercury and sodium lights
- Fuse panels
- Water and gas pipelines with associated 'net' currents
- Uninterrupted power supplies (UPS)
- Hearing-aid induction loops
- Room fans
- Electronic medical procedures, especially MRI scans
- Daylight
- Weather changes
- Laser beams in supermarkets

- Thyristors, systems used to control power in appliances such as vacuum cleaners
- Signalling circuits for cable TV
- Geopathic stress – disturbances in the Earth's fields.

So it is clear that if you find yourself becoming ill around a number of these sources, you will need to take some kind of action.

What you can do

Untreated EHS is a serious public health concern, and the number of people suffering from this condition is growing. Yet diagnosis can be very difficult. As we've seen, EHS is not yet recognised as a specific medical condition. GPs often lack information about it, and some are downright sceptical. EHS cannot be directly improved by most medication, so this may have an effect on whether it is recognised, as drug companies do not see a way of making a profit from it.

The problem is compounded because people with EHS often cannot go into hospital for tests using high-tech equipment. This may be unbearable for the person with EHS.

What you will find is that having EHS is a bit like developing diabetes. Life can never be the same again. There is no magic wand that can enable you to go back to your previous way of life without risking a reoccurrence of the symptoms.

With EHS, you have to pay very careful attention to your environment because it can contain invisible hazards that you have to predict, where possible, and against which you need to take avoiding action.

We list below the ways you can reduce your exposure, and some treatment possibilities that have helped improve the symptoms of some people with EHS. We have also included rarer solutions tried by some people with EHS – sometimes in desperation when the medical profession have let them down. The difficulty is that not everything works for everybody, so it is a matter of trying what has worked for others to see if it will also help you.

It may seem obvious, but the most important change for you to make, in the opinion of many who have EHS, is to avoid EMFs as much as you can. Let's see how to make that as easy as possible for you.

Reducing exposure at home

Below we describe the electrical appliances, computers, and so on that people with EHS report most frequently as provoking their symptoms. Chapters 4 and 5 cover other appliances and EMF sources. Follow the advice given in those chapters, but remember that if you suffer from EHS you have to be further away and take more precautions than people without the condition.

Electric appliances – general

☺ **Unplug electric appliances** when not in use. The cables from the socket to the appliance still produce electric fields even when the appliance is switched off.

Computer monitors

🗑 It is important to remember that monitors give off higher fields to the side and the back, **so keep your distance**. Even low-emission monitors can provoke symptoms in people with EHS.

☺ The display on your PC computer monitor is refreshed many times every second. The Windows default setting is usually 60 Hz (times per second). It is a good idea to **change this rate**. In our experience it is unwise to have a vertical refresh rate slower than 72 or faster than 100 times a second, as more people report eye strain and headaches outside of this range.

🗑 EHS can be initiated by an exposure to chemicals. Computer monitors, and many other electronic items, give off quite toxic volatile organic chemicals (VOCs) when the cases and electronic components are first turned on. If possible, leave the computer and monitor fully working 24 hours a day in a well-ventilated, unoccupied room for a couple of weeks before you start to use it. This can help, but the offending chemicals can continue to be 'outgassed' for six months or more.

🗑 Work carried out at Bristol University has shown that the static electric field generated by monitors and TV screens can attract negatively charged particles to the screen and positively charged particles in the opposite direction – towards the user. These particles may include chemicals that can trigger or perpetuate EHS symptoms. **Keep your screens clean**.

☺ A **negative ioniser** may help you feel better in this atmosphere. Be careful in your purchase of a negative ioniser, as some contain a cheap transformer that can give off high electromagnetic fields nearby. We have researched and found one that we believe to be excellent (available from EMFields).

☺ **Good ventilation** is important – air the room well during the day and have a window or ventilator slightly open at night.

Laptop computers

🗑 Laptop computers are usually worse than PCs, most being unearthed and giving off enormous powerfrequency electric fields. It is important that you **earth a laptop** computer, or run it off batteries.

🗑 Some people with EHS react to laptops and flat desktop screens because they can emit significant levels of radio-frequency electric fields from the back illumination and scanning processes. The TCO and MPRII standards governing PCs specify limits up to 10 times lower for these higher frequencies (see Chapter 4).

To work on his computer, Peter has to keep it over 2 metres away and have a data projector screen for the computer and a mouse that uses infrared. He has a keyboard that has an infrared connection with the computer and is battery powered, with a range of 3 metres. He says it looks like most of these are being discontinued but a Google search for 'infrared keyboard airkey' finds a selection.

He has replaced standard network cables with shielded ones.

Televisions

🗑 Some EHS (and ME) sufferers find their symptoms are made worse when watching television. It is not clear what causes this. Mrs Jones, who is highly EHS, was really keen to watch digital TV when most horse racing was transferred to a 'digital only' channel. Despite trying several digital TVs she was unable to find one that did not bring on her EHS symptoms, but after switching back to her analogue TV the symptoms greatly decreased. It is possible that it was the chemical vapours (VOCs) being given off by the new digital TVs that were the problem rather than the really low levels of EMFs we found.

☺ The ME society suggest that if TVs are a problem for you, do not sit between the television set and the aerial. You should sit so that you face the television and the aerial is also in front of you, however it is mounted. We see no technical reason why this should reduce the symptoms people suffer from, but it worked for a sufferer from severe EHS whom we know, who had tried everything else. Anyway, moving the TV, seat or aerial is worth a try.

Telephones

🗑 🗑 🗑 Radiofrequency emissions from mobile phones and cordless phones can allow in **toxic chemicals** that would normally be kept out of the brain by the 'blood-brain barrier'. Once this happens the chemicals may interfere with the way cells are working, leading to peripheral neuropathy (stinging, burning pain, numbness, tingling and prickling of extremities), which is reported by many people who have EHS.

?? You may begin to react not only to mobile phones and DECT phones, but also to **ordinary wired phones**.

?? Some people have bought **speakerphones** in order to increase the distance between themselves and the equipment. This can work well, but only if the equipment is earthed – many speakerphones are not. They are usually not as clear as ordinary phones, which can make conversations more difficult.

☺ **Low-EMF phones** can be seen on www.teloray.se. They are CE-marked – that is, tested and approved for use throughout the EU. The company, TeLoRay Systems, allow a trial period of one month.

See Chapter 3 for a full discussion of telephones.

Wiring

If you have EHS, it is important to remember that you need to be more aware of house wiring than the majority of people and take precautionary measures if you're to avoid adverse health consequences. Chapter 4 covers home wiring in more detail. Remember that all wiring needs to be done by a 'competent person' according to the IEE and the Part P Building Regulations.

☺ We recommend **radial ('tree and branch') wiring** and, ideally, that all mains electricity wiring is run in **earthed metal conduit** or pipes, as was the practice 50 years ago. This almost completely removes the electric field inside the house. If not, then we recommend the use of screened cable.

☺ **'Demand switches'** (see Chapter 4) installed next to the main consumer unit (fuse box) can be useful to reduce night-time EMFs dramatically when rewiring isn't a possibility. This is only any use if you can use separate circuitry for equipment such as fridges, freezers and air conditioning, which need to work all night.

☺ **Using foil to reduce electric fields**
Earthed aluminium foil will reduce electric fields from wiring, whether the wires run underneath floorboards or inside walls. You can use ordinary supermarket aluminium foil: it is cheap and easily available. Be aware that you will need to take up

your carpet or flooring and redecorate your walls afterwards.

When doing your floor, it's best to do the entire area. Once you've taken up the carpet lay the strips of foil so they overlap by about 5 cm. Alternate the way you lay the strips, with the first shiny side up, the second shiny side down, and so on. Hold the strips in place using ordinary sticky tape (such as Sellotape) and connect to the electricity earth in one place using a wire leading to an earthed water pipe or to the earth pin of an ordinary mains plug that should then be inserted into an electrical socket. Re-cover with the carpet or flooring.

You can use foil on the walls in the same way, alternating the strips as above. As plaster is often very slightly porous, the electrical field can 'leak' into the walls from sockets and cables, causing high fields across large sections. Foil can reduce exposure to this as well as to incoming microwave fields (such as those from mobile phone masts). You can paper over the strips of foil, using wallpaper, or lining paper and good quality wallpaper paste that can then be painted. The foil should be earthed as described above.

One problem with earthed foil is that it attracts electric fields, so if you haven't covered up the source, the fields can actually increase. As a result, it's often necessary to do both walls and floor.

Special conductive paint (see EMFields) is now available, which is easier to use, enables walls to breathe and is non-toxic. It can be overpainted with ordinary emulsion.

Lighting

☺ You might consider installing **direct current (DC) lighting circuits**. These give off zero pulsing EMFs and are much less likely to provoke adverse health reactions. They are not readily available at the point of writing and Powerwatch can advise on the latest situation.

🗑 You should **avoid all electronic room light dimmer switches**.

🗑 **Fluorescent lighting** is problematic for people with EHS, but it's unclear which aspect of it they are reacting to. Various hypotheses have linked EHS to EMFs from the transformers in the tube fixtures, the 'flicker' of the light and the spectrum of light.

🗑 Even the better modern fluorescent lights, with electronic high-frequency ballasts, give off higher EMFs than an equivalent old-fashioned incandescent bulb. So while they are useful for power-saving in hallways and rooms where the light is on for long periods, we do not recommend them for use in desk or bedside lights.

Reducing your exposure from appliances

DO

✔ Unplug appliances when not in use.

✔ Keep your distance from the back and sides of a computer monitor.

✔ Make sure the vertical refresh rate on your computer monitor is between 72 and 100 times a second.

✔ Let a new monitor 'run in' in an empty room for a couple of weeks before you begin to use it.

✔ Earth your laptop computer, or run it off batteries.

✔ Keep the monitor screen clean using an anti-static cloth.

✔ Improve the atmosphere of a room containing a

computer with a negative ioniser.

✔ Make sure the TV set and its aerial are both in front of you.

✔ Do not use a mobile or digital cordless phone, except in emergencies.

✔ Use ordinary incandescent bulbs wherever possible.

Reducing your exposure from wiring and lighting

DO

✔ If wiring or rewiring a property, use radial wiring.

✔ All wires ideally should be run in conduit (metal pipes), or, if not practicable, use screened cable.

✔ If rewiring is not practicable, try installing a demand switch on appropriate circuits.

✔ If your electric fields are high near the wall, use aluminium foil or conductive paint on the walls and the floor to screen the radiation.

✔ Consider installing DC lighting.

DON'T

✗ Don't use electronic dimmer switches.

✗ Don't use fluorescent lights close to you.

Making other changes in the home

Chemicals

Many people who are electrically sensitive are also sensitive to chemicals to a varying degree. In fact, EHS can actually be triggered by chemical exposure. So if you have EHS, or suspect that you do, try to avoid exposure to chemicals, wherever practicable.

🗑 🗑 🗑

These days, a staggering array of **household chemicals** fill the average under-sink cupboard. Those you may develop sensitivity to include household cleaners; garden chemicals; wood treatment; pest treatment; fresh paint and solvents, which release toxic compounds; new carpeting and vinyl flooring, which may release hormone-disrupting chemicals; treated wooden floors and furniture, which give off formaldehyde; building materials; newsprint; perfumes; and hair perming solutions.

According to GreenHealthWatch (see Resources), in 2000, UK householders spent £35 million on pesticides for their houses and gardens (39 per cent up on 1999 spending). Public gardens, parks and playing fields are also heavily treated with pesticides. Friends of the Earth revealed that monitoring by the government showed that residues regularly exceed acceptable safety levels.

Nor is the countryside any greener. In 2004, the chief executive of the UK Countryside Agency announced in a speech that 500 types of chemicals are routinely used in conventional farming and more than 25,000 tonnes of pesticides are used each year in the UK, which imported over 3 million tonnes of synthetic fertilisers last year from over 40 different countries.

☺ NASA has researched the ability of different **plants to detoxify the air**, reported in B.C. Wolverton's *Eco-Friendly House Plants* (see Further Reading).

According to NASA, many easy-to-grow houseplants such as spider plants, Boston ferns and peace lilies are excellent for cleansing the air of formaldehyde and other chemicals in small quantities. Microbes in the roots biodegrade the pollutants into chemicals that can be used as a source of food for the microbes and the plant itself.

Peace lilies, for instance, excel at removing bioeffluents such as carbon monoxide, hydrogen, methane, alcohols, phenols, methyl indole, aldehydes, ammonia, hydrogen sulphide, volatile fatty acids, indol, mercaptans and nitrogen oxides, which are emitted through normal biological processes by people simply being in a room. Plants in a room also release phytochemicals that suppress mould spores and bacteria by up to 60 per cent more than occurs in a room with no plants. An added benefit of Boston and other ferns is that they thrive in areas of low light, which doesn't confine them to windowsills and allows you to place them where you need them to do the job.

🗑 A **freshly painted nursery**, complete with new carpeting, a cot, mattresses, blankets, clothing and toys is a room that is likely to be high in chemical emissions unless ecological paints and natural materials (not treated for stain resistance!) are used.

Windows

🗑 **Metal-framed windows** (including aluminium framing used in double glazing) can resonate at microwave frequencies and amplify the signals coming into a room. If you react to radiofrequency EMFs, this may not be the best type of window frame to have installed.

☺ **Pilkington-K double glazing units**, designed for good thermal insulation, have one inner surface coated with a thin metallic film. They offer a reasonable level of protection against incoming radiofrequency radiation, stopping over 99 per cent of microwaves from 300 to 3000 MHz. This glass is mandatory in double glazing put into new buildings. As far as we know, it is not available as single glazing, nor is it mandatory in replacement windows, though all double glazing firms will stock it. If it is available as a single pane, you would have to be very careful with cleaning it, as scratches may begin to let in microwaves.

Furniture

☺ **Furniture** and furnishings should ideally be made of **natural materials** to avoid the build-up of electrostatic charge. Central heating and inadequate humidity or ventilation resulting in a dry atmosphere can make static electricity worse.

Furniture treated with cellulose and silicone-based furniture finishes, when rubbed with polishing rags and dusters, often produces a high positive charge. Use natural wax finishes wherever possible.

🗑 Ideally ensure that neither your **bedframe** nor your **mattress** has **metal parts**. These can pick up mains frequency fields and microwave radiation and also distort the earth's DC fields in major ways. There is some evidence that this can be bad for your health. Wooden bedframes and futons are alternatives, but you may need to search to find the kinds that are suitable for your posture and comfort requirements.

🗑 🗑 Most **electrically adjustable beds** have transformers that give off high EMFs even when you are not adjusting them. We do not recommend this kind of bed if you have EHS.

Making changes at work

Chapter 5 contains detailed information about EMF exposure in the working environment.

?? If you suffer from EHS, it would be useful to get your employer or union representative to carry out an **EMF survey** of your working environment. You might then become involved in making recommendations for any remedial work that's necessary.

☺ Meanwhile, **take breaks outside** where possible. This earths electrostatic fields and replenishes negative ions.

☺ **Work in natural light and in well-ventilated areas** wherever possible. Keep air-conditioning systems clean and well maintained. Keep the ambient temperature as cool as you can manage. Warmth breeds bacteria, which can further impair a vulnerable immune system.

☺ Keep your working environment as **free from dust** as possible. Reduce the amount of chemicals in the environment, including cleaning materials used.

The insurance company Skandia, in Sweden, is one of several companies that have reorganised their electrical systems at work. This has resulted in a dramatic reduction in people calling in sick. 300 employees had symptoms prior to the reorganisation of the electrical systems and other measures. Today, no employees are sick due to hypersensitivity to electricity, and the company has established a purchasing policy for display screens and electrical apparatus.

Making changes in the home . . .

DO

✔ Reduce the amount of chemicals you use in the house and garden.

✔ Think carefully before installing new window frames. You should consider installing double glazing units that use Pilkington-K glass.

✔ Buy some houseplants to help detoxify the house.

✔ Buy furniture made of natural materials wherever possible. Choose a natural wax finish for wood.

✔ Ensure adequate ventilation and level of humidity.

✔ Reduce the amount of metal in your bed.

DON'T

✗ Do not have carpets and furniture treated with 'stain resistant' finishes before purchase.

. . . and at work

DO

✔ Ask your employer to do a full EMF survey.

✔ Take regular breaks from work, preferably outside.

✔ Work in natural light and good ventilation wherever possible.

DON'T

✗ Do not use more chemicals than absolutely necessary to keep your work environment clean.

Personal changes

What you wear

☺ If you have EHS, you should wear **clothes and shoes** made of **natural materials**. You might even consider buying special anti-static clothing and footwear made for workers in the electronics semiconductor industry.

☺ You need to have flooring made of natural material, as you build up static charges every time you move your feet. You should **'earth' yourself frequently** by touching metal objects, or walking barefoot on the ground outside.

☺ To **prevent a build-up of potentially harmful ions**, it has been suggested that when you come home from work you should promptly remove your shoes and walk around in bare feet or wear socks or slippers of natural materials.

☺ One ME sufferer who was desperate to find any way she could to improve her symptoms found that her continuous migraine-type headaches were entirely eliminated when she started **wearing glasses with all-plastic frames** instead of metal ones. She thinks that the metal frames may have been 'picking up' electrical or other forms of radiated fields.

🗑 **Metal necklaces, chains and arm bangles should only be worn with care** as they form a conductive loop than can capture and amplify some frequencies (depending on their length and shape) of EMFs. If you really want to wear them we suggest you have a plastic connector inserted so that the metal does not make a complete loop, but we suggest you don't wear them at all if you have EHS.

Grounding or earthing

All electrical fields and charges want to 'return home' to where they came from – ultimately this usually means the 'Ground' or the earth. Our mains electricity systems are connected to the earth at regular intervals in the electricity distribution network. In our house wiring, one wire (the 'neutral') of the 230 volts supply is connected to the earth back at the electricity substation.

This means that all electric fields coming from electrical wiring and appliances are trying to get back to earth, and the natural electrical conductivity of your body is the means by which it often tries to do this. One way to prevent the fields returning to earth through people is to provide a **better** path to earth close to the wiring or appliance. Hence the idea of screened wiring (or metal conduit) discussed in chapter 4. Static electricity can also affect sensitive people. To avoid this problem, we suggest that you only wear natural materials and, if still necessary, you can 'earth' yourself.

☺ The best thing to do is to remove or screen house wiring, thus eliminating the EMFs at their source.

☺ **Earthing straps and kits** are available. An earthing strap is one way you can maintain an earth bond so that your body does not become 'charged up' (but see below for our caution).

☺ One way of making your own earthing link is by attaching a wire to ground from a bracelet. made of copper or other conductive material. This will restrict the distance you can move while you are wearing the link, but some EHS people have reported that it has helped them a lot.

☺ One person found that a length of copper tube knocked 3 feet into the ground, with a wire attached, greatly reduced her symptoms when she held the wire indoors.

WARNING

🗑 **There is an important cautionary point regarding this kind of 'personal earthing' via copper tubing and a wire.**

● **It is important to avoid sitting near any electrical equipment when you 'are earthed'. The electric fields generated by the house wiring and equipment will seek out the easiest path to earth, and you are likely to become this.**

Diet

🗑 It is unclear what effect eating **genetically modified food** may have on our immune systems. Volunteers who ate one meal containing genetically modified soya had traces of the modified bacteria in their small intestines.[41] If gastric problems are one of the symptoms of your sensitivity, it is worth being extra vigilant and avoiding GM foods whenever possible. Some scientists now fear that the antibiotic resistance genes often inserted into GM crops as markers – which allow genetic engineers to see whether the traits they have inserted have 'taken' – will leave us completely vulnerable to new variant diseases. The worry is that the resistance genes will transfer to disease-causing bacteria.

☺ Wherever possible, **eat plenty of fruit and vegetables**, organically and locally produced and in season. Eat as little processed food as is practicable. Eating the best-quality whole-foods you can get is not a new idea and is recommended as part of most diets for better nutrition and health. To quote Richard Wakeford, the Countryside Agency's Chief Executive, on 23 June 2004, '*Over the last sixty years there has been a decline in trace elements in fruit and vegetables; calcium content is down by 46%; copper by 75%; carrots have lost 75% of their magnesium and broccoli has lost 75% of its calcium.*' It is believed that this is a result of intensive farming practices and plant breeding for appearance on supermarket shelves. Offsetting this reduction by only eating top-quality produce has never been more important.

▯ It is often worthwhile to **monitor your general diet** closely. Skin sensitivity (including reddening, as an allergic-type reaction to EMF exposure) may be alleviated by reducing your intake of some fish and wines, which contain histamine, and the celery family, which contains skin sensitisers.

☺ The amino acid tryptophan is necessary in your diet for your body to be able to make melatonin. Tryptophan is found in turkey, cottage cheese, oats, bananas and eggs. Melatonin is the hormone involved in improving the immune system, fighting cancer and stabilising moods. It is primarily produced at night, so if you are hungry in the evening, try a tryptophan-rich snack. And sleep in a dark room – this is very important.

?? Have a trace element test (your GP can arrange this). If you have EHS you may be low in zinc, copper, selenium and magnesium – all essentials for well-being and healthy functioning of mind and body. Supplements are not always taken up by the body very efficiently, and it's worth finding out what foods are rich in the elements you are short of and increasing them in your diet. There are many books specifically about diet, trace elements and supplements that you could consult for further information.

Water

🗑 Some pollutants, or relatively new additives to drinking water like fluoride, may be predisposing people to EHS either directly or via a general weakening of the immune system.

🗑 Most people suffer from a degree of subclinical dehydration. (Feeling tired is a symptom of subclinical dehydration. Feeling thirsty is a symptom of extreme dehydration.) This is because tea and coffee contain diuretics, so you excrete more liquid than you take in. The body needs considerable quantities of water to function effectively. It is much better to drink water, herbal teas or water-based squash.

☺ A man should drink 2 litres of still (not fizzy) water and a woman, $1^1/_2$ litres.

☺ As an addition to this, try a hypoallergenic moisturising cream. It helps with skin rehydration, may improve any problems you may have with dry skin and can help to reduce EHS symptoms.

☺ If you are electrically and chemically sensitive, it is important to filter your drinking water. In many areas, underground water pipe supplies are run in parallel with electricity supplies, which some people claim results in the water being homeopathically imprinted by 50 Hz. Work by Jacques Benveniste, and others, have shown that homeopathic remedies can both be created and damaged by electromagnetic fields.[42] Putting a small permanent magnet underneath the filter jug should help remove this. If you use an electric kettle to boil water you intend to drink, you should also place the small magnet underneath the mug or cup for a couple of minutes to remove powerfrequency imprinting effects induced by the electric current in the heating element. See Resources section for obtaining suitable magnets.

🗑 If you decide to **filter** your incoming water supply, do not use a unit with reverse osmosis filters. These result in 'hungry' water which will leach minerals necessary for health from your bones and other body tissues, which you will then excrete in urine.

Supplements

☺ **MSM** (methylsulfonylmethane, a form of organic sulphur) is considered by some to be a food. Norman Shealy, inventor of the TENS machine and founding president of the American Holistic Medical Association, reports that taken in doses of a gram or so daily, MSM will increase levels of the beneficial compound dihydroxyepiandrosterone (DHEA) dramatically in about 50 per cent of patients.

DHEA has anti-aging and anti-cancer properties. It is present in high levels in brain tissue and is known to enhance the body's general immune response. DHEA levels are known to decrease precipitously with age, falling 90 per cent in the period between the ages of 20 and 90. People with clinical depression have been found to have low levels of DHEA.

☺ **Vitamin C** taken along with MSM increases the level of DHEA in about 70 per cent or so of people. Together with vitamin E, vitamin C increases protection against membrane damage from free radicals. MSM and vitamin C also help reduce arthritis symptoms in many people.

Although not specifically tested for people with EHS, MSM seems to be helpful in combating some of the symptoms commonly found as part of this syndrome. There are no known side effects, except that sulphur turns silver jewellery you may be wearing black within about a week.

Alasdair had been having osteopathy for back problems over some months. He embarked on a course of MSM and his osteopath said, 'I don't know what you've been doing, but your bones and muscles feel as supple as if you were 20 years younger.' He continues to take it and believes that 1 gram of MSM and the same of slow-release vitamin C each day is worth trying if you have any EHS symptoms. It seems to help many people with EHS, but a few have reported it makes them feel worse. You will know how it will affect you within about two weeks of starting to take this combination daily.

☺ **Evening primrose oil and starflower oil** provide essential fatty acids which can help with conditions involving a generalised allergic reaction.

☺ Sleep disturbance is one of the symptoms experienced by people suffering from EHS, especially those who react to mobile phone mast radiation. A dietary supplement that seems to be effective is Mellodyn, a proprietary combination of extracts of the herbs valerian, chamomile, passion flower and lemon balm with melatonin.

Reducing exposure through personal changes

DO

✔ Wear clothes and shoes made of natural materials.

✔ 'Earth' yourself regularly by touching a radiator or other metal object.

✔ You might want to try wearing plastic rather than metal-framed glasses.

✔ Try to avoid wearing metal necklaces or bracelets.

✔ Eat lots of fresh fruit and vegetables, local and in season, ideally, and unprocessed food, generally.

✔ Have a tryptophan-rich snack in the evening. Eat foods rich in trace elements you may be short of.

✔ Men should drink 2 litres of water a day and women $1^1/_2$ litres, in addition to any tea, coffee, cola or alcohol, which are diuretics.

✔ Use a hypoallergenic moisturising cream regularly to rehydrate your skin.

✔ Take a course of MSM and vitamin C and monitor any changes.

✔ Evening primrose oil may help boost your immune system.

✔ Mellodyn may improve sleeping patterns.

DON'T

✘ Avoid GM food.

✘ Avoid histamine-containing foods.

✘ Do not use a reverse osmosis filter to filter your water supply.

Treatments

A number of treatments have helped people with EHS, ranging
from the allopathic to the homoeopathic and into the realm of
healing. We list the ones that we or others have found work
the best. As we are all unique, you may need to try more than
one approach or treatment before you arrive at one that alleviates your symptoms.

- **Chiropractic** has proved helpful in cases where
  EHS has been triggered by trauma, especially to
  the back and neck.
- **Osteopathy** has apparently helped the immune
  system of some people with EHS. Cranial
  osteopathy may also improve cerebrospinal fluid
  flow in the cranium.
- Some **homoeopathic remedies** have been devised
  specially for people who have EHS. One EHS
  sufferer found that homoeopathy helped her cope
  with severe pain; another, who also has ME, has
  found that the homoeopathic dose of belladonna
  helps her balance. Your local homoeopath may be
  unfamiliar with the particular remedies concerned,
  but can contact the Homoeopathic Association for
  further information. In the UK, Dr Jean Monro of
  the Breakspear Hospital in Hemel Hempstead and
  Dr David Dowson, a complementary medicine
  specialist practising in Bath and London, also
  prescribe for the electrically hypersensitive. (See
  Resources for contact details.)

▯ Homoeopathic remedies become **useless near high EMFs**,
and lose all their potentisation. Be careful where you put them,
and avoid placing them near magnets, including loudspeaker
magnets, and do not put them near to the wheels of cars or

trains you're travelling in. Using homoeopathic remedies will not help as much if the environment you live and/or work in remains at a toxic EMF level.

- Several environmental medicine practitioners cite **provocation/neutralisation testing** – a form of immunotherapy – as a key element in the treatment of both EHS and multiple chemical sensitivity (MCS). This is an unorthodox technique and is not recognised by most medical doctors. A signal generator some distance from the patient is used to find the frequency that will trigger the allergic reaction. Then other frequencies are tested to find the neutralising frequencies that stop the reaction. Signals at these frequencies can 'potentise' vials of water that can be carried by the patient and used to stop the reaction, which they do by holding the vial of water in their hand. (See Further Reading: Oschman and Smith & Best)
- **Neurontin** (gabapentin), a prescription drug based on an enzyme used to treat epilepsy and some neuralgias, has been used in the US for treating EHS symptoms. Alasdair, who was prescribed this drug for trigeminal neuralgia (a nerve pain), has also found that it significantly reduces his electrical sensitivity. Several EHS people who have tried Neurontin report a lessening of EHS reaction symptoms, especially when they are related to chemical and food sensitivities.

  Dr Jay Seastrunk of Dallas, Texas, uses Neurontin to help people with environmental illnesses. He claims that the treatment does not merely mask symptoms but rather helps to quiet inflamed cells/tissues and prevent further damage.

Interestingly, the drug works partly by changing the electrical activity of cells.

An effective dose is 1500 to 2100 mg per day, which is approximately double the dose for epilepsy. It has few recorded side effects, although it only seems to help some EHS sufferers.

- Sleeping on several different geopathic stress lines are implicated in the development of serious illness, including cancer and CFS. The edge line of an underground stream is associated with increasing the susceptibility of biological systems to EMF radiation. You could dowse where you sleep to ensure that your bed is not on one of the earth energy lines associated with ill health, and move your bed if this is the case. Roy Riggs (see Resources) carries out EMF and geopathic stress house surveys in the UK.
- Healers and spiritual healers. We have had some good reports on the effects of healing on people suffering with EHS. Sometimes it eliminates symptoms entirely and sometimes ameliorates them significantly. Prayer has also been found to be effective, as is the case in most instances of ill health.

Other possibilities

The following are suggestions that have helped at least one person with EHS that we have heard from. They will not all work for everyone, but if you feel you would like to try one or some of the ideas below, they are very unlikely to make matters worse and could well help you. Many of them may not offer immediate relief, so it can be worth persevering.

We would be very happy to hear of your personal experiences with any of these suggestions, or to make further ones that have worked for you, that we can pass on to others. Email us at info@emfields.org (see Resources).

- Acupuncture.
- Reflexology. It relieved the EHS symptoms in someone who also suffers from ME.
- Magnet therapy. One person with EHS and ME found relief from mobile phone mast-induced fibromyalgia by using magnets.
- Promazin helped an EHS sufferer cope with the pain she experienced when exposed to EMFs. This drug is also prescribed for radiation sickness, though it is not in common use.
- Salt and baking soda, used in a number of ways, as follows:

1. 2 tablespoons of Epsom salts in a bag carried around in places of exposure really helps some people.
2. A salt and baking soda bath (using 2 cups of each) is soothing when you are feeling 'zapped', 'fried' or 'electrified'. It is unclear why the bath has this effect but it eases the distress, possibly because it changes the skin's conductivity level. It may well be a good idea to use a hypoallergenic moisturising lotion afterwards to keep the skin moist.
3. For acute relief of facial symptoms, try some sea salt and baking soda in a bowl used for about a minute as a face wash. Again, it may well be a good idea to use a hypoallergenic moisturising lotion afterwards.

- Baths or drinks using green therapeutic clay may reduce symptoms or restore energy. (See Resouces)
- Cactuses can be useful in a room where a computer is in use, as the spines, which have sharp points, will attract charged aerosols and clean the air. It is a good idea to rinse them occasionally and put them outside for a while during the day when the weather is warm enough. So keep more than one to circulate them. Always have good ventilation so that there are adequate numbers of negative ions in the air.
- A number of Oriental disciplines have had a positive effect for some EHS patients. One is Qi Gong. There is clearly some kind of interaction with the immune system going on here, the dynamics of which are, as yet, poorly understood. One person finds practising Aikido three times a week helps. Tai chi has been found found to increase memory T cells (a type of immune cell) by 50 per cent when practised for 45 minutes three days a week for 15 weeks.[43]

It is important to remember that lifestyle changes which improve the immune system or which affect the subtle energy systems of the body are going to have much less impact if you do not remove the source of EMFs responsible for your EHS. This needs to be tracked down at the same time, and the necessary changes made.

Other protection devices?

🗑 Many devices (such as medallions, buttons, 'towers', mains plug-in 'stress neutralisers', stick-on gizmos, and so on) are available on the market that *claim* to help protect against or neutralise the EMF/ELF or other output from electrical appliances such as computers, and microwave sources such as mobile phones. With most of the products we have seen there is no scientific foundation for their claims and some we have examined in detail can only be described as useless 'snake-oil' scam products. The pseudo-scientific literature that is associated with the products is usually flawed and completely useless. The only thing you can be sure of is that the manufacturers see a market for the device that will create money for them.

?? There is a possibility that *some* of these devices may have a very subtle effect on the body's immune system, and help the person using the device to be able to repair the damage that has been done by EMFs, by improving their immune function, once they have eliminated the EMF source. However, the effect is likely to be very subtle and at the moment we do not have the scientific instruments to measure such changes in body dynamics. The 'protection devices' certainly do not eliminate or remove the source of the potential damage, which is still verifiably present.

We suggest that if you are tempted to try any of these devices, obtain it on a money-back if not satisfied arrangement. If it works for you, keep it; if it doesn't, return it.

Psychological approaches

In 2003 Dr Robert Coghill of the Wake Forest University School of Medicine in Winston-Salem, North Carolina, tested the pain sensitivity of 17 healthy volunteers normally, and when they were in MRI brain scanners.

Coghill found that the scans showed very different responses depending on whether the volunteers had previously expressed the ability to bear pain. The thalamus, which receives pain messages from the spinal cord and peripheral nerves, was active in all 17 participants. Those least able to bear pain showed more activity in the cerebral cortex, associated with higher cognitive function.

In 2003, Professor Norbert Leitgeb and colleagues at the Technical University of Graz showed that people with EHS had a higher level of cortical arousal, as well as other physiological differences, than people without the condition.[44] Coghill's conclusion was that for people with EHS, pain was not dampened en route to the brain, so all the differences must be due to the way the cerebral cortex interprets the information based on prior experience. People suffering from EHS may be 'conditioned' to respond far more strongly to stimuli than other people, following the sensitisation of parts of the brain from some as yet unidentified electro-biochemical signal.

For the sensitised individual, it may be useful to find ways of desensitising past experiences in order to learn new techniques of managing incoming stimuli. Some of the differences in interpreting incoming data may be genetically determined, but some will be learned and thus capable of being unlearned or relearned. This may be why in some experiments people report on the effectiveness of placebos as well as 'real' treatments.

☺ Hypnotherapy, meditation, and other 'psychological' techniques have been found to be effective.

☺ Techniques for stress management are extremely useful because stress makes symptoms worse.

☺ Cognitive behavioural therapy (CBT) may have beneficial effects in some people with EHS. Various studies[45] have shown mixed results, but it could be worth a try. It is currently being

promoted as the best 'orthodox' treatment for idiopathic problems including EHS.

☺ There are other, innovative ways of alleviating the symptoms of difficult-to-treat syndromes. Here is an interesting
example.

A group of people with allergies were asked to come off all
allergy medication for three days before watching the Charlie
Chaplin film, *Modern Times*. Before, during and after the film
they were exposed to various allergy-causing substances.

Their allergic responses were significantly reduced after
watching the film. But when the same experiment was tried
with a group of people watching a weather forecast, no
improvements were detected.[46]

Scientists believe that laughter stimulates the production of
endorphins, chemicals which give us a 'high' and also boost
the immune system. Laughter – even the anticipation of
laughter – shifts our internal chemistry measurably, reducing
stress hormones and increasing the number of natural virus-
killer cells available to fight diseases from colds to cancer (see
Martha Beck's *The Joy Diet*, 2003). The amount of time we
spend laughing appears to shrink as we get older. The average
6-year-old laughs 300 times a day, compared to a grouchy 47
laughs a day in adulthood. Women generally laugh more than
men. We are unsure how the researchers determined how
often the average person laughs, but you may be aware of
where on the laughter spectrum you would put yourself. See if
there are ways you can bring more laughs into your life, if you
realise you're lacking in them.

☺ Listening to music you love encourages a profound and
positive emotional experience which, in turn, stimulates the

body's production of hormones and chemicals which protect against disease. Students who sing in a school choir or play musical instruments tend to do better all round (see Don Campbell's *The Mozart Effect*, 1997).

There are no magical cures for EHS, but following the suggestions above, you should be able to make a significant difference to the limiting effect of the symptoms. Some of the ideas on offer might even make your life more fun.

It is important to catch EHS as early as possible. The longer you have been suffering the symptoms, the longer it is likely to take to reduce them.

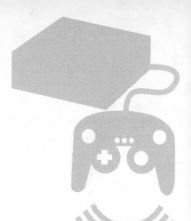

Appendix: Making Sense of the Science

Electromagnetic fields are necessary for life. But in certain circumstances, they may also be a potential carcinogen as well as a trigger for other illnesses and conditions. In this appendix, we look at the scientific evidence for this link.

We believe that the published evidence so far already shows that EMF exposure increases the risk of cancer and a range of degenerative diseases and psychological problems that may well be passed on to future generations.

Moreover, we feel that mobile phones – which irradiate our heads with both pulsing microwaves and low frequency fields – may well turn out to be one of the most devastating long-term self-harming acts of mankind. Our greatest fear, which we discuss later, is that this practice will cause an epidemic of early-onset dementia in our children.

Safe or dangerous?

Journalists and the public alike often expect science to tell them whether something is 'safe' or 'dangerous' (though both are value judgements), and get frustrated and confused when senior scientists completely disagree with each other. They ask how politicians can protect us when even the scientists are failing to agree among themselves. Of course, neither the science nor the politics are anywhere near as simple as such questioning assumes.

So you may read: 'Under certain conditions EMFs may cause you physical or psychological harm.' Which is ambiguous enough; but the subtext is often something like, 'We can't admit there is a problem unless someone is prepared to pay for preventative measures.'

Research into the way EMFs affect our bodies, known as bioelectromagnetics, is seriously challenging conventional wisdom in biology, neurology, the physical sciences and engineering. Since the first reports of physiological responses to low levels of EMF exposure appeared over 35 years ago, there has been ongoing fierce and dismissive opposition from scientists holding orthodox views and from industries fearing 'unreasonable' restrictions being placed on their activities.

In the context of EMFs' effects on human health, there are probably several hundred thousand relevant scientific studies and 10,000 very relevant ones. To attempt to evaluate and discuss these in a book such as this would not be appropriate or possible.

So here is our methodology. We read the conclusions of groups of respected scientists who have published literature reviews (and tell you how you can get their reports), and include the results of other important studies. Generally, we find the conclusions of the official literature reviews too vague and weak to be very helpful, but they can still be useful source documents. We come to our conclusions based on the science they have collected together and what else we have read and thought about for the last 20 years. We also look at what scientists call 'anecdotal' or 'grey' (non-peer-reviewed) evidence and add our views. We will provide you with some important historical perspective on the issues of public health and safety, science and protection.

Public health, public perceptions

At the time of writing this, the beginning of 2006, there is far more scientific evidence regarding the dangers associated with EMF exposure (at power, radio and microwave frequencies) than there is of those associated with passive smoking. So why is there such a difference in official attitudes to the need for precaution? The history of smoking can be revealing in this context.

Tobacco was probably first brought to Britain in the 16th century, and in 1856 the first UK cigarette factory opened in London. A year earlier *The Lancet*, the British medical journal, had started a serious debate they dubbed 'The Great Tobacco Question: Is Smoking Injurious to Health?' However, by 1900, cigarettes were a part of normal life for many people and sales were raising significant taxes for governments.[47]

In 1950, researchers reported that 'prolonged use of tobacco seems to be an important factor in the induction of bronchio-genic carcinoma', that lung cancer is rare in non-smoking males, and that there could be a lag of 10 years or more 'between the cessation of smoking tobacco and the occurrence of clinical symptoms of cancer'.[48] In this year, Richard Doll and Bradford Hill also presented their preliminary report on smoking and lung cancer,[49] followed by their major one in 1952.[50]

Twelve years later, in 1964, the US government officially recognised that smoking caused lung cancer and the UK government banned cigarette advertising on television and later brought in cigarette packet health warning labels. Yet one top UK government medical official told Alasdair over lunch in the early 1990s that 'people get pleasure and the extra taxes more than pay for smoking-related public health-care costs. Smokers generally live ten years less than non-smokers, thus reducing pension payments and saving the government large sums of money.'

Yet in 2000, smoking was directly responsible for 5 million painful, premature deaths worldwide, or about 12 per cent of all deaths each year. The World Health Organization estimates that by 2030, more than 10 million people will die around the world every year from smoking-related diseases. Since 2000, public outcry has forced some governments to act more decisively, with some countries starting to ban smoking in public places.

So – leaving out *The Lancet*'s prescient question of 1855 – it took about 14 years from the first sure evidence that smoking is harmful to any official governmental recognition that it is. With radiation safety and petrochemical safety issues, the process seems to have taken about 75 years, from when health problems were first reported to when formal government action to adequately protect the public was begun.[51]

In the 1980s, along came the mobile communications industry with a product that apparently wasn't polluting or dangerous to health. The mobile phone companies needed operating licences that earned governments many tens of billions of pounds, euros or dollars. There is also a regular monthly tax income from all the mobile phone calls that are made.

In 2004, the UK's mobile telecommunications turnover was £55.9 billion, of which retail revenues were £47.4 billion (6 per cent higher than in 2003), forming 4.1 per cent of the country's GDP. This boom is wonderful for industry, commerce and governments. Inevitably, not one of them wants to see the industry upset by extra regulations. And one speculates that even advice to users that mobile phone use might be giving them long-term health problems would not be welcome either.

Why do we think this? You have only to hark back to the BSE crisis. In February 1988, 15 months after the first cow was diagnosed with BSE, UK civil servants recommended that the government introduce a slaughter and compensation policy for clinically diseased cattle which would only have cost a few million pounds.

The UK agriculture minister John MacGregor rejected that advice in 1988. His private secretary explained why: 'He (the Minister) does not see how we could proceed without it being clear where the offsetting savings are coming from . . . '.[52] Due to a lack of action, the total cost of BSE to the UK taxpayer is set to top £4 billion – over 1,000 times more.[53]

We believe that similar considerations are now delaying necessary precautionary action to reduce human exposure to EMFs.

A new take on biology?

Dr Bruce Lipton, an internationally recognised cell biologist and one of the pioneers of the new branch of science called epigenetics, wrote that 'Conventional medical researchers have no understanding of the molecular mechanisms that truly provide for life.'[54]

We believe that damning statement to be true and it is one of the main reasons why so little progress has been made in investigating the interactions between EMFs and humans or animals.

The current training our clinicians undergo places the emphasis on dealing with physical and psychological problems via drug prescription, surgery or perhaps psychotherapy. Medics are happy enough to accept the use of modern diagnostic techniques such as MRI and CT or CAT scans, which rely on your body reacting to the EMFs given off by the machine – without ever realising that our bodies also react to background EMF pollution.

Most of us, including medical researchers, still think that more of something will produce a bigger effect – a phenomenon known as the 'dose-response' relationship. In fact, living systems often do not react in that way, and they do so only rarely at the molecular level. Small electrical charges and signals play an enormous part in life processes, including DNA winding and unwinding, where very weak (non-ionising) forces guide the copying process.

Life is dependent on water. When a baby is born it is about 78 per cent water, falling to 50 to 65 per cent in adult life. The way hydrogen and oxygen atoms bond together means that all water molecules are magnetically charged, allowing them to 'align' themselves with environmental magnetic fields.

One of Alasdair's early experiments in 1971 was to design and make a proton magnetometer. This consisted of a bottle containing water around which a coil was wound. By passing an electric current through the coil a large magnetic field is created that aligns all the water molecules in one direction. When the current is turned off, the water molecules realign themselves with the Earth's magnetic field. By measuring the frequency that the water molecules emit as they do this we are able to determine the local geomagnetic field to about one part in a million. This demonstrates the magnetic sensitivity of water molecules, which we all mainly consist of.

Now, in the 21st century, we are surrounded by EMFs – and these are very likely to react with our bodies.

When we encounter a 1 microtesla 50Hz EMF, for example from an electric cooker or hairdryer, (and remember, the official safe limits for exposure are up to 100 microtesla in our homes – and more at work), it will physically affect the water in our bodies 50 times every second. Does this matter? Maybe, maybe not, but let us clearly understand that water and other molecules in our body and our body cells *do* react to it. If we expose them directly to low-frequency fields (from 10 Hz to about 1000 Hz), then, at certain frequencies, we see clear changes in the normal functioning of the cells that may reduce our well-being.[55]

Conventional scientists often state that they know of no mechanism whereby the cells in our bodies can process electromagnetic signals. In fact, the conventional biological science that they hang on to cannot even yet explain the amazing human and animal sensitivities to light, sound, taste or smell.

To take a well-proven example, the hearing threshold of a healthy young person involves the vibration of part of the inner ear of only 0.00000000001 (10^{-11}) metres, or about the diameter of a single hydrogen atom. The cells in the ear somehow collectively (co-operatively) suppress the vastly larger internal molecular noise, by an as yet unknown mechanism, and function as an almost perfect amplifier. We do not yet understand just how living biological systems can have a considerably better performance than advanced modern electronic circuits.[56]

In traditional science, organisms are thought not to react to an energy stimulus unless it exceeds the background environmental noise level. Traditional EMF biological science assumes that anything under the background 'noise' level would have no effect, yet there are now thousands of scientific studies showing that this is not the case. There are plenty of experiments in the literature that 'show no effect', but that does not mean you can dismiss the ones that do.

Beyond the molecule

The quantum view of the universe reveals a complex web of atomic interactions and communications. More than 40 years ago, the renowned Nobel Prize-winning physiologist Albert Szent-Gyorgyi published a book called *Introduction to a Submolecular Biology*.[57] He attempted to bring an awareness of the importance of quantum physics in biological systems to life scientists. His peers considered the book to be the ravings of a once brilliant but now senile old man, and took little notice.

Yet Professor Frank Weinhold, writing in the respected science journal *Nature* in May 2001, notes that organic chemistry provides the mechanistic foundation for biomedicine but is so far out of date that its textbooks still had not incorporated quantum mechanics.[58] He asks the question: 'What are the forces that control the twisting and folding of molecules into complex shapes?' Weinhold believes they are electromagnetic and probably mainly electric at the molecular level. If this is true, it is no wonder that exposure to EMFs can affect your health.

Many hundreds of scientific studies over the last 50 years have revealed that the 'invisible forces' of the electromagnetic spectrum have a profound impact on biological regulation in our bodies. These forces range from extremely low-frequency natural geophysical forces through to EMFs from our many uses of electricity, radio and microwaves. There is even evidence of the effects of a newly recognised, but not yet widely accepted, theoretical force – scalar energy. These forces influence cellular behaviour that contributes to the unfolding of life.

Dr Bruce Lipton[59] writes: 'Though these quantum effects research studies have been published in some of the most respected mainstream biomedical journals, their revolutionary findings have not been incorporated into the medical school curriculum.'

The full complexity of living biological organisms is far from understood and scientists are still a long way from knowing what life is – what gives the 'spark' of life to inanimate matter.

Our genome – or total genetic composition – is like a recipe book that can both photocopy and read itself. Conventional science accepts that it unwinds and winds up again using very weak electromagnetic forces. It is transcribed into messenger RNA and then converted into strings of amino acids that fold up into proteins.

Changes in this folding and so in the final shape of the molecules are one of the repeatedly reported effects of EMF exposure, and are known to be influenced by electric charges. Almost everything in our bodies is either made of proteins, or made by proteins. Every protein is a translated gene. Both single- and double-strand DNA breaks have been shown to become more common when living cells are exposed to quite low levels of man-made EMFs.

This is our premise. Now let's look at the different types of EMFs and their possible effects on the human body.

Powerfrequency EMFs

Powerfrequency electric and magnetic fields – that is, EMFs at 50 to 60 Hz – surround us. They're produced in varying degrees and strengths by all parts of the electricity supply system, from high-voltage powerlines to the electrical appliances and wiring in our homes. As we've seen, EMFs have come under scrutiny as a possible source of harm and have been blamed for a wide range of adverse health effects. A great deal of research has been carried out investigating these possible effects, with mixed results.

The difficulties for researchers

Those mixed results could be down to several factors. There is some evidence, for example, that we all have different sensitivities to EMFs. If 10 per cent of the population were susceptible to EMF-related effects and maybe 20 per cent of these were exposed enough to be affected, then the 2 cases per 100 would be most unlikely to show up in a normal whole population study.

Another possible problem is that we are all exposed and affected. This means that there are no people who can be used as the 'control' comparison group.

In 1998, Sam Milham reanalysed the data assembled by the late Richard Doll, who conclusively established the link between smoking and lung cancer,[60] which showed that the odds ratio for heavy smokers was 23.7 (that is, they were 23.7 times more likely to die from lung cancer than nonsmokers). Milham found that when you compare the figures for heavy smokers with moderate ones, the odds ratio falls to 1.9,[61] because moderate smokers already have an elevated risk. In other words, if you can't find an unexposed population, then the odds ratios will be quite small.

Sam Milham found some evidence that the rise in incidence of childhood leukaemia may be associated with electrification. The peak which occurs among 2- to 5-year-olds did not exist prior to the widespread electrification of the US in the 1920s and rural leukaemias followed electrification.[62] It is almost impossible to find a population in developed countries that is not exposed to electricity. Many studies have now shown an increased risk of childhood leukaemia with EMF exposure in the range 1.5 to 2-fold. These low ORs are often dismissed as too low to matter but they are similar to those for smoking.

This underlines our point that assessing EMF exposure is problematic because everyone is exposed to a degree. At a National Radiological Protection Board public meeting in May 1999, Alasdair asked Sir Richard Doll about this problem. He replied: 'Yes, for EMFs we do not have any unexposed and very few highly exposed people, so odds ratios are likely to be quite low.' A low odds ratio for large numbers of people would represent a very considerable public health problem.

The debate among scientists

The early debate over EMFs and health is covered well in books by Robert Becker, Paul Brodeur and Cyril Smith (see Further Reading).

By 1972, Soviet researchers had linked EMFs with low-grade health problems such as fatigue and headaches. In 1977, Becker, a physician, and biophysicist Andrew Marino, testified before the New York State Public Service Commission about the results of their experiment, which showed negative health effects due to exposure to extremely low-frequency EMFs.

But the debate really hotted up with the publication of Nancy Wertheimer and Ed Leeper's paper linking childhood leukaemia with EMFs[63] (see Chapter 1).

The 1989–1993 US National Council on Radiation Protection and Measurement (NCRP) Scientific Committee spent some years looking at the available information, and by 1995 had produced a draft report. This committee was made up of eminent and well-regarded scientists who understood very well the areas of research they were evaluating. Their draft report had some highly precautionary recommendations aiming for maximum residential levels of 0.2 microtesla (magnetic field) and 10 volts per metre (electric field).[64] But the 800-page draft report was never finally published and was effectively suppressed by the US government and industry (documented in various issues of *Microwave News*). However, the NCRP allowed the epidemiology section to be published as Chapter 7 in the second edition of the *Handbook of Biological Effects of Electromagnetic Fields.*[65]

This stated that the weight of evidence supported an association of childhood leukaemia with proximity to powerlines, and an increased risk of leukaemia and brain tumours associated with occupational EMF exposure. Other possible cancer associations are plausible based on laboratory research on melatonin. These include breast cancer in women and prostate cancer in men.

By the late 1990s, funding for powerfrequency health-related research in the US virtually dried up. Most EMF bio-effect researchers had to switch to investigating other things.

The childhood leukaemia link

Perhaps the largest body of evidence relates to childhood leukaemia, as we've seen. The bulk of it comes from epidemiological studies that have looked at the pattern of childhood leukaemia in relation to levels of exposure to EMF. Since the first study was published in 1979, more than 25 epidemiological studies around the world have investigated the association between childhood leukaemia and exposure to EMF. Most of the individual studies were unable to prove or disprove the link as they were limited by the relative rarity of childhood leukaemia and further by the relatively low number of children exposed to higher levels of EMF.

A number of researchers have now done meta-analyses, bringing together data collected from the individual studies.[66]

Anders Ahlbom and Sander Greenland reported an approximate doubling of the incidence of childhood leukaemia at 0.4 microtesla. Daniel Wartenberg reported a lower odds ratio of 1.3, but concluded that the effect was relatively consistent and may have contributed 15 to 25 per cent of childhood leukaemia cases. In 2004, Michinori Kabuto and his colleagues found that children exposed to these levels had close to five times the expected rate of leukaemia.[67]

At the CHILDREN with LEUKAEMIA conference at which this was reported, Ahlbom said that there was probably a leukaemia risk below 0.4 microtesla because, in his opinion, it is unlikely that there is a threshold for the EMF effect.[68] This is a significant comment from someone who is known to be cautious and who has been studying EMFs and childhood leukaemia for 20 years.

The largest epidemiological study of childhood leukaemia and powerlines was recently published in the *British Medical*

Journal.[69] The authors reported an increased risk of leukaemia in children in England and Wales whose birth address fell within 600 metres of a high-voltage powerline. Around 150 metres from lines, the risk was nearly double the norm.

The incidence of childhood leukaemia went up in the UK,[70] 19 European countries[71] and the US[72] by over 60 per cent between 1950 and 2000, an increase of about 1 per cent per year, and a fivefold rise during the 20th century.

Various causes have been put forward and natural ionising radiation probably accounts for about 30 per cent of cases. This ionising exposure is generally being reduced by improved measures lowering the levels of naturally occurring radon gas in houses. Chemicals in our environment are blamed by some people. The strongest contender for the bulk of cases, which occur in the age range from 2 to 5 years of age, is EMF exposure, to the child *in utero* as well as after birth.

One possible cause is the effect of corona ions emitted by high-voltage overhead powerlines. These charge up toxic aerosols, effectively making them more likely to get into your bloodstream when breathed in.[73] This could partly explain the effects found up to 600 metres away in the Draper report[74] – a distance too far away to be magnetic fields, as they are back to below 0.4 microtesla by 100 or 150 metres. Electric fields have been implicated in a number of other papers, so we believe that human exposure to electric fields should be minimised.[75] In Dr Anthony Miller's Ontario Hydro adult worker study, when they took only magnetic fields into account, the increased risk of developing leukaemia was 1.6. When they looked at electric fields it was similar. However, when they looked at workers exposed to electric **and** magnetic fields, the risk rose to 11.2 times that of unexposed workers.

EMFs and other illnesses

There is good evidence that EMFs play a role in the development of brain and breast cancer,[76] miscarriages,[77] depression and suicide,[78] Alzheimer's[79] and ALS or Lou Gehrig's disease, a form of motor-neurone disease.[80]

Taking a precautionary approach

There are well-established mechanisms by which EMFs *could* produce biological effects, but results from many hundreds of research projects since 1979 are contradictory and inconclusive.

Exposure to powerfrequency EMFs has been shown to damage DNA, to alter cell function and accelerate tumour development. However, for each study that shows an effect, there are good and reproducible studies that show no effect. This presents difficulties for the scientific community, and there is still considerable controversy among the scientists working in this area.

One relatively firm finding is a genetic (heritable) tendency to be susceptible to EMFs. This was first clearly shown for chickens and then for other animals. Individual cell lines may also show such differences – which in turn may have an effect on the results of experiments.

The World Health Organization discourages health officials at the national level from setting, as a precautionary measure, stricter guideline levels than the official ICNIRP guidelines for protecting populations. As we have already seen, the current limit endorsed by the WHO is 100 microtesla, even though childhood leukaemia is internationally linked to exposure levels of 0.4 microtesla (250 times lower), and the International Agency for Research on Cancer (IARC) classified EMFs in 2001 as a possible human carcinogen, prompting a vigorous debate over whether it should be in the 'probable' class.

Michael Kundi of the University of Vienna says that applying the same guidelines as the WHO uses for air pollutants to EMFs would lead to an exposure limit of 0.2 microtesla – 500 times lower than the current UK limit. This is explained in his conference paper.[81]

The biological proof is not there – yet. When it is, as we believe will happen, the time for legislation will arrive.

Pandora's box – radiofrequency and microwaves

Artificial microwave and radiofrequency radiation are new environmental pollutants, dating back only a few decades. As the WHO said in 1981:

> The rapid proliferation of such sources and the substantial increase in radiation levels is likely to produce 'electromagnetic pollution' . . . Problems of pollution range from electromagnetic interference, particularly in relation to the operation of health services, to direct risks to the health of individuals.

Since then, concern about RF and microwaves has continued to grow, prompting the WHO to set up its EMF Project in 1996. The project's website states:

> Electromagnetic fields of all frequencies represent one of the most common and fastest growing environmental influences, about which anxiety and speculation are spreading. All populations are now exposed

to varying degrees of EMF, and the levels will
continue to increase as technology advances.

Our exposure to man-made sources of microwave and RF radiation is now many orders of magnitude higher than that from
natural radiation. Humans as a species have had no opportun-
ity to adapt to such high environmental RF levels. As we've
seen, the responses of different organisms to this form of radiation can differ, as can responses from individual to individual
and within one individual over time. Some of us, for example
people with allergies, react to lower levels of pollutants. All this
needs to be taken into account when setting exposure guidance levels.

The emerging picture

Over the years it has become increasingly clear that electromagnetic fields (both at mains frequency and radiofrequency)
are not as safe as they were first thought.

In the US as long ago as 1948, a possible link between
microwaves and testicular degeneration in dogs was reported. A
1953 study of workers at Hughes Aircraft Corporation found
excessive amounts of internal bleeding, leukaemia, cataracts,
headaches, brain tumours, heart conditions, and other problems
in employees working with radar, a form of pulsed RF radiation.

The first significant report describing occupational 'microwave
sickness' appeared in 1974.[82] This syndrome includes fatigue,
headaches, palpitations, insomnia, skin symptoms, impotence
and altered blood pressure.

The prominent American epidemiologist Charlotte Silverman
also described 'microwave sickness' due to low levels of exposure to EMFs in 1979[83] – the same year that Nancy

Wertheimer and Ed Leeper published their seminal paper linking childhood leukaemia to magnetic fields from our use of electricity (see Chapter 1).

Increasingly, as modern telecommunications has developed, the public has become more continuously exposed to levels of pulsing microwave radiation that only workers previously experienced from time to time. The general public is now complaining of the symptoms of microwave sickness.

In 1996, the European Commission Expert Group, then chaired by the UK National Radiological Protection Board's Dr Alastair McKinlay,[84] was mandated to draw up a blueprint for research into possible health effects relating to the use of mobile telephone technology. At the end of that year it gave a report recommending a €24 million research programme. The report stated:

> A large number of biological effects have been reported in cell cultures and in animals, often in response to exposure to relatively low-level fields, which are not well established but which may have health implications and are, hence, the subject of ongoing research . . . A substantial body of data exists describing biological responses to AM RF (including microwave) fields at SARs [specific absorption rates of radiation] too low to involve any response to heating. It has been suggested that non-equilibrium processes are significant in the bioenergetics of living systems, challenging the traditional approach of equi-librium thermodynamics.

The ongoing European Co-operation in the Field of Scientific and Technical Research (COST) programme, including the

COST244bis Report[85] and the COST 281[86] activities, confirm the EC's continuing concern about these matters.

In December 1997, after a WHO scientific meeting, the head of the WHO EMF Project told a news conference that perceived risks from new technologies have become a serious public health issue:

> Mobile phones have only been around for less than 10 years now and the incubation period for cancer is at least 10, maybe 15 years. So we need to set up the studies so that if there is an impact, it can be found in a reasonable time.

You should note that the World Health Organization definition of 'adverse health effects' include those affecting a person's 'well-being' and includes headaches, unusual fatigue and sleep disruption.

Professor William Leiss, an eminent Canadian expert in environmental risk management, said in reply: 'The public might be excused for thinking that ordinary citizens differ from rats chiefly in that the latter are used in short-term experiments and the former in longer-term ones.'[87]

In 1998, the WHO started to admit that there were adverse biological effects caused by exposure to RF fields, but refused to admit that they might damage human health:

> Exposure to low levels of RF fields, too low to produce heating, has been reported to alter the electrical activity of the brain in cats and rabbits by changing calcium ion mobility. This effect has also been reported in isolated tissues and cells. Other studies have suggested that RF fields change the

proliferation rate of cells, alter enzyme activity or affect the genes in the DNA of cells. However, these effects are not well established, nor are their implications for human health sufficiently well understood to provide a basis for restricting human exposure.[88]

To give you some idea of the scale of these things and the large differences in opinion as to what levels may be 'safe', Table A1 compares natural levels with typical and allowed human exposure at cellular phone frequencies. The figures are approximate as the actual levels vary with frequency. Units are microwatts per square centimetre.

Table A1 – RF Power level comparisons[89]

(microwatts per square centimetre)

cosmic radiation, 1000 MHz	0.0000000000000001
natural background, all RF frequencies	0.0000000001
from one cellular satellite	0.0000001
Median level 15 US cities, 1977	0.005 *FM radio & TV*
Schwarzenburg sleep disturbance from	0.001
Salzburg guidance at house windows 2002	0.001 (0.02 V/m) max
Salzburg maximum guidance level 1998	0.1 (0.6 V/m)
Skrunda children adverse health effects	1.0
100 metres from cellular base station	1.0 (2 V/m)
can regularly be found up to	10 (6 V/m)

Some maximum guidance levels:

Switzerland, Lichtenstein, Luxembourg	10	(6 V/m)
Italy, Russia, PRChina	10	(6 V/m)
ICNIRP, UK, EU, etc, USA similar	1,000 allowed public levels!	

More recently, in March 2001, the then chairman of the Independent Expert Group on Mobile Phones (IEGMP), Sir William Stewart, gave oral evidence to a recent UK Trade and Industry Select Committee Inquiry,[90] including this comment:

> It is simply not possible to say that there are no potential effects on the human population. It is difficult to talk about the population because populations vary. Antibiotics do a wonderful job for the general population, but there is a subgroup in the population that is allergic to antibiotics; they cannot take them. There is a sub-group in the general population who cannot eat nuts because they are allergic to them. That is why we refer to the general population. The other point is that we mentioned health effects and well-being effects. On the basis of discussions such as those we came to advise on the need for a precautionary approach.

The REFLEX project, which looked at the effects of low-level RF radiation on cellular systems, was carried out by 12 research groups in seven European countries. Their report[91] has made a substantial contribution to the known biological effects of EMFs on cells *in vitro* (that is, in a laboratory cell-culture dish).

The project's researchers found changes in numerous genes and proteins after exposing living cells *in vitro* to EMFs at levels well below current international safety guidance. Gene mutations and inappropriate cell activity were found, for instance. The study concluded that this kind of damage is real, and that it is important to carry out much more research, especially focusing on the monitoring of people's long-term health. The lead researcher, Franz Adlkofer of the Verum Foundation, advised against using mobile phones when fixed line phones are available and also recommended using a headset (hands-free kit) with a mobile phone whenever possible.

The research into mobiles

Both users' reports, and ongoing research, reveal much to be concerned about when it comes to mobile phones.

We saw some of the serious diseases and other conditions linked to mobile phone use in Chapter 3. Many users also report dizzy spells, fatigue, headaches, loss of concentration, memory loss and confusion, skin irritation, tingling or burning, twitching, eye 'tics', buzzing in their head at night. The confusion and memory loss are very similar to symptoms of dementia.

The memory loss connection

Professor Henry Lai's team[92] in Seattle, Washington, in the US have found that exposure to radiation from mobile phones seems to cause memory loss in rats. The rats seemed unable to remember how to get to their food after an hour's microwave exposure. RF/microwave radiation at a frequency of 2450 MHz has been found to alter the effect of benzodiazepines, such as Valium.

Lai concluded that since benzodiazepine receptors are found in most regions of the brain, and can undergo changes after brief exposure to radiation, urgent investigations into such interactions should be funded. More than 12 years later, this work has still not been done with humans.

The blood-brain barrier link

Dr Leif Salford and colleagues at Lund University in Sweden meanwhile claim mobile phone users could be at risk of

developing Alzheimer's disease, multiple sclerosis and
Parkinson's disease.

His team exposed rats to microwave fields which, mimicking
GSM mobile phone emissions, were not strong enough to heat
up brain tissue. Only two hours of exposure disabled the
blood-brain barrier – which normally protects the brain from
toxins – allowing proteins to enter the brain. Salford's team
found clear evidence of significant brain-cell death following
the pulsed microwave exposure. Alzheimer's and MS are both
linked to abnormal proteins in the brain. Salford and his team
fear that mobile phone use is likely to cause premature onset
of illnesses linked to ageing, particularly among teenagers, who
are heavy mobile users.[93]

During an interview on the UK's BBC Radio 4 *You and Yours*
programme, on 5 February 2003, Salford said he would not
allow his children to use a mobile phone other than in a real
emergency and he chooses not to use one other than when he
really has to. He added that he rated the reality of long-term
brain damage as a 'probability rather than a possibility'.

Salford's work on the blood-brain barrier confirms studies
carried out over the last 35 years. Early Soviet microwave radiation research was documented in the 1976 *American
Defense Intelligence Agency Document*, DST-1810S-074076.
Since declassification there have been a number of new
versions of this document, with increasing numbers of
censored pages. In 1998, when a campaigner in Northern
Ireland applied for a copy of this document as evidence in the
battle against mobile phone masts in schools, she was sent a
sheaf of virtually blank pages. The uncensored document,
however, reveals that Soviet military scientists had successfully
used microwaves of the type emitted by mobile phones to
weaken the blood-brain barrier.

According to Dr Louis Slesin, editor of the American specialist journal *Microwave News*, US Army scientists had succeeded in duplicating the Soviet experiments by 1977 – eight years before mobile phones became generally available in Britain.[94] However, mobile phone users have been told repeatedly by the industry and by government-funded bodies that there is no credible scientific evidence that mobiles can cause harmful effects.

Dr Allan Frey, working with American military funding, carried out some of the earliest research into microwave irradiation effects on humans in the 1960s. His continued work led him to believe that there is 'significant evidence' of adverse health effects as a result of using mobile phones.[95]

Meanwhile, Professor Darius Leszczynski's team at the Finnish Radiation and Nuclear Safety Authority reported in June 2002 that exposing human cells to one hour of mobile phone radiation triggered a response which normally only occurs when cells are being damaged, allowing tiny molecules to pass through the blood-brain barrier into brain tissue. He said, 'If this were to occur repeatedly over a long period of time, it might cause brain tissue damage.'

Leszczynski went on: 'We need further studies looking at real people to see if the blood-brain barrier is affected . . . If it does happen it could lead to disturbances, such as headaches, feeling tired or problems with sleeping.' He added, 'What I believe is that we will find these leaks occur in humans.'[96]

Sir William Stewart, now chairman of the UK Health Protection Agency, said this research by Leszczynski should be taken seriously because it came from 'a well-respected team at a well-respected institution'. However, Dr Michael Clark, scientific spokesman at the (then) UK National Radiological Protection

Board, commented: 'It is important work and part of the jigsaw to see whether mobile phone radiation really has any health effect, but we need to remember that all sorts of things – tea, caffeine, red wine, sugar – have biological effects without necessarily damaging health.'[97] A remark that we believe does not help move the debate forward.

Children and mobiles

Other researchers have focused on the effect of microwave radiation from mobile phones on children. Professor Om Gandhi at the University of Utah found that five-year-old children soak up 50 per cent more radiation than adults during a mobile phone call.[98] Their thin skulls, thinner ears and smaller heads offer less protection against microwaves sent out by the phones. As a result, there is potentially a far greater risk of damage to their brain cells. Brain activity in children who use mobile phones for as little as two minutes can be altered.

In a small unpublished study, Dr Michael Klieeisen from the Neuro Diagnostic Research Institute in Marbella, Spain, found that a single call lasting just two minutes can alter the natural electrical activity of a child's brain for up to an hour afterwards. It was also found that the microwaves penetrated deep into the brain and not just around the ear. Klieeisen tested one 11-year-old and a 13-year-old using a CATEEM scanner linked to a machine measuring brain wave activity. His team was able to make photographic images of the changes in brain electrical activity.[99]

Professor Sianette Kwee of the University of Aarhus, Denmark, and a participant in the European Union's COST 281 project, 'Potential health effects from emerging wireless communication systems', reports:

Our studies showed that there was a significant change in cell growth in human amnion cells after being exposed to EMF fields from both power lines (ELF) and from mobile phones (MW). These biological effects were greatest in young and vigorously growing cells. These results tell us, that e.g. microwave fields from mobile phones can be expected to affect children to a much higher degree than adults.[100]

Dr Staffan Edström, a professor in tumour surgery at the Sahlgrenska Hospital in Gothenburg, Sweden, has linked radiation from mobile phones with the increase in oral cancer among the young.[101] Since then, dentists in the UK have reported an increase in oral cancer incidence in teenagers.

In September 2001 the Russian non-ionising radiation and health committee stated that pregnant women and children under 16 years of age should not use a mobile phone. They also recommended limiting the duration of mobile phone calls to a maximum of three minutes, and allowing a period between calls of a minimum of 15 minutes with the preferred use of headsets and hands-free systems.[102]

The brain tumour trail
The evidence is becoming stronger that increased mobile phone use over time significantly raises the risk of developing brain tumours. For two leading researchers into EMFs and health at least, the research itself has been a rough road.

Professors Ross Adey and Henry Lai revealed in May 1999 that multinational companies had tried to influence the results of their research into mobile phone effects.

Adey, a biologist, said he had had his funding withdrawn by Motorola before completing research showing that mobile phone emissions affected the number of brain tumours in animals. Meanwhile Lai, who has been studying the biological effects of electromagnetic fields for 20 years, was asked three times to change his findings on how such fields caused genetic damage in rats. And when Dr Jerry Phillips published his experiments, which supported Lai's experiments, his contract with Motorola was terminated. Dr George Carlo, who had headed up the $25M Cellular Telephone Industry's Wireless Telephone Research EMF health programme, bitterly criticised the industry for failing to act on his findings and for not taking safety matters seriously.[103]

Another obstacle in clarifying the link between brain tumours and mobile phone use, is the nature of the disease. Most brain tumours are very slow-growing, and few are diagnosed before 10 years have elapsed from the time the cancer took hold. Some take up to 30 years to be diagnosed. So it is most unlikely that any study would find a significant change in incidence levels before at least a decade had passed.

That said, there does seem to be a significant increase in benign brain tumours, malignant astrocytomas, and acoustic neuromas – a rare form of benign tumour – in people who have used a mobile phone or cordless phone for over five years, which increases after 10 years use.[104] But it is likely that it will be at least 2015 before the link becomes clear.

The media has widely and incorrectly reported that the published parts of the largest-ever study ('Interphone') into mobile phone use and brain cancer showed no increase in brain tumours after the first 10 years of use.[105] In fact, these studies did find an increasing risk over time after 5 years. This misreporting seems to have been generated by the misleading press releases circulated by the researchers. We believe that this is a deliberate distortion of the truth for unknown reasons.

Effect on brain waves

Various eminent researchers have shown changes in brain activity, including electrical activity as measured by an EEG, after exposure to mobile phone frequencies. Lebrecht Von Klitzing also researched the effects of cordless DECT telephones on human brainwave patterns. After five minutes' exposure, he found changes in brainwave activity and blood flow.[106]

Dr Alexander Borbely and his team at the Neuroscience Center in Zurich found that exposure to a digital mobile phone signal altered sleep and brainwave patterns.[107] Volunteers exposed to 15-minute periods of emissions from mobile phones spent less time awake during the night, and the electrical patterns shown by EEG varied by up to 15 per cent. This finding has now been replicated by an Australian group.[108]

Dr Ray Tice and Graham Hook, of Integrated Laboratory Systems in North Carolina, found serious changes in human blood cells following exposure to four different types of cellphone signals.[109] The nuclei of many red blood cells had been split into little bits known as micronuclei – direct evidence of genetic damage to the cells. This was a well-controlled and repeated set of experiments that showed a two- to eightfold increase in micronuclei in the blood after exposure to cellphone-type microwave radiation for 24 hours. The relationship between the presence of micronuclei and cancer is so strong that doctors around the world use tests for micronuclei to identify patients likely to develop cancer.

Exposure to masts

In most residential areas, aside from cordless phones and mobile phone handsets, it's the signals from mobile phone masts that are the dominant radiofrequency signals. These differ in 'quality' from FM radio and TV broadcasts in that almost all mobile phone systems emit bursts of pulses.[110] As we have seen, it's the pulsing nature of these new signals that most concerns leading bio-effects scientists. This is a very new phenomenon in health epidemiology terms – and when you recall that most cancers and chronic debilitating conditions take many years to develop, we simply do not know where it's leading us.

It's also important to note that there has been very little epidemiological research published in respected journals that evaluates the symptoms of people living near mobile phone masts, although the evidence that does exist seems to confirm anecdotal evidence that the health of nearby residents is affected in a substantial minority of the population. Let's look at some of these cases now.

Leukaemia and other cancers

A study of 128,000 Polish military personnel over 15 years found that about 3,700 of them were considered to be occu-pationally exposed to RF and microwave radiation of around 5 to 10 $\mu W/cm^2$ (4 to 6 V/m) – levels that can be found near some mobile phone base stations.[111] This exposed group had something like a tenfold increased risk of developing adult chronic leukaemia, and were found to be six times more likely to develop non-Hodgkin's lymphomas (NHL). NHL is one of the most rapidly increasing types of cancer. Between 1973 and 1997, incidence grew in the U.S. by 81%.[112]

In north Sydney, Australia, Dr Bruce Hocking found almost a doubling of childhood leukaemia within a 4-kilometre radius of the area's three TV towers.[113] Of the 123 cases of leukaemia diagnosed from 1972–93, it was found that there was a 55 per cent chance of survival for five years among those living in areas closest to the towers. In areas further away, the figure was 71 per cent. Hocking concluded that 'there was an association between proximity to the TV towers and decreased survival, among cases of childhood leukaemia'. He published a follow-up study four years later.[114]

Investigating reports from a local doctor, Helen Dolk of the London School of Hygiene and Tropical Medicine found an increase in a range of cancers around the large Sutton Coldfield TV and radio transmitter.[115] Publication was held back for a couple of years while they extended the study to other broadcast transmitters. A similar-sized increase was not found in this follow-up study, though there were some increases in cancers.

A report by German doctors on a group of 1,000 patients in the town of Naila showed a threefold increased risk of cancer in those living within 400 metres of a base station, when compared to people living further away.[116] Measured RF fields showed a threshold of about 0.05 V/m, above which increasing levels of health problems were reported by the doctors' patients.

A number of studies have now indicated that this surprisingly low level of pulsing microwaves seems to be the signal strength above which increasing adverse health problems are reported.

In Israel, two local doctors studied a small community for a year, and found that living within 350 metres of a 10-metre-high mobile phone mast led to a fourfold increase in cancer in the general population and a tenfold increase for women.[117]

The same number of cancers were diagnosed in this area in the year following the study as were diagnosed in the year of study. These cancers developed quite quickly, indicating a potentially strong promotional effect of the RF emissions, which were typically well below 1 V/m.

Loss of concentration and other disorders

In 1995 in Schwarzenburg, Switzerland, near shortwave masts, Ekkehardt Altpeter and colleagues at the University of Berne found adverse health effects such as anxiety, restlessness, sleep disruption, joint pains, decreased concentration, and general weakness and tiredness, in the local community.[118] They found a dose-response relationship with sleep disturbance at levels above 0.001 μW/cm^2. Switzerland has now closed the mast down, and the government allows only very low exposure levels of radiofrequency for the general public.

A study in Latvia by Russian researchers looked at 966 children living near a pulsed RF military station at Skrunda.[119] They found that motor function, memory and attention were significantly worse in the exposed group, and their neuro-muscular endurance was decreased. They also found a sixfold increase in chromosomal damage in exposed cows had occurred at exposure levels below 6 V/m.

In October 2003, a Spanish study found a significant correlation between the declared severity of a range of adverse health symptoms and the measured microwave signal strength from masts transmitting at 1800 MHz.[120] The separation of the local residents into two different groups depending on their level of exposure also showed an increase of the declared severity in the group with the higher exposure. Mobile phone and personal computer usage were low in both groups.

When Dr Gerd Oberfeld of Salzburg's Public Health Department in Austria did a follow-up analysis of this Spanish study, he found statistically significant exposure-response associations for a number of conditions: fatigue, irritability, headaches, nausea, loss of appetite, sleep disorder, depressive tendency, feeling of discomfort, difficulty in concentration, loss of memory, visual disorder, dizziness and cardiovascular problems.[121]

The analysis showed a fifty-nine-fold increase in depression, a fortyfold increase in fatigue and a twentyfold increase in concentration problems in people living in measured GSM (global system for mobile communications) field strengths between 0.25–1.3 V/m, when compared with people living in field strengths below 0.05 V/m. Most of the symptoms found by Oberfeld also appeared in an analysis of 530 people living near masts in France by Professor Santini of the University of Lyons.[122]

A government-funded Dutch study by Professor Peter Zwamborn was prompted after people living near a base station reported to the country's health monitoring network that they were suffering adverse health effects.[123] A healthy control group was found to make up a larger group of about 76. When both groups were exposed to 3G base station signals under short-term test conditions, both suffered. Cognitive functions such as memory and response times were affected, as well as headaches and nausea.

Interviewed on the BBC Radio 4 *You and Yours* programme in 2003, Zwamborn said the study had been expected to confirm that there were no effects at low signal levels (1 V/m) but that they had found significant adverse effects on 'well-being'.

There have also been reports that both mobile phones and radio masts cause an increased incidence of epileptic seizures.

One anecdotal report states that a policeman brought a TETRA handset home and placed it on the table. His young, healthy son pressed 'transmit' and had an instant epileptic seizure – and he had never had one before. There have been various documented instances of more seizures occurring near base stations (see www.tetrawatch.net).

We are now being exposed to higher frequencies than this, including vehicle anti-collision radar (61–100 GHz) and tera-hertz (THz, 1,000–20,000 GHz) whole body imaging (for medical and security purposes). The THz-Bridge project has reported both genotoxic and epigenetic effects induced in human lymphocytes following exposure to 100 GHz radiation 100 times lower than the ICNIRP guidelines.[124]

Recent official viewpoints:

- The International Commission on Non-Ionizing Radiation Protection has issued an epidemiology overview.[125]

We believe that this ignores most of the most relevant recent reports of ill health related to microwave exposure, especially regarding exposure from mobile phone base stations.

- In 2004, the NRPB issued a general *Review of the Scientific Evidence*.[126]

This contains some useful comments on some of the science but reaches no useful conclusions as far as the protection of the public is concerned.

- The UK's National Radiation Protection Board (NRPB) issued an update[127] of the original *Stewart Report*.[128]

The Board of the NRPB should be commended for producing this extra report. It was a vast improvement in terms of public health concern on the earlier 2004 review and offers some guidance about practical aspects of public exposure to microwave emissions and their possible effect on health. It makes a number of practical precautionary suggestions for progressing this difficult issue.

- The latest World Health Organization views can be found on their EMF Project website.[129]

This website contains a curious mix of statements calling for a precautionary approach and then immediately sidesteps them with conclusions that no precautionary action needs to be taken at present.

It is worth remembering that the worldwide boom in mobile phones has created a tension between the desire for profits and the need to protect public health.

What we need to do

We feel that based on the now robust findings on the link between EMFs and childhood leukaemia, and increasing evidence of links with other cancers and disorders, it is time for governments to take action.

Studies identifying vulnerable subgroups are important, rather than focusing on whole population studies in which meaningful data about sub-groups gets lost. This is particularly important as regards people who are electrically sensitive.

The minimum action regarding mains frequency EMF exposure should be:

- A moratorium on new building close to powerlines and electricity substations
- High-voltage powerlines should be undergrounded (keeping away from homes) where possible
- Public Guidance should be issued on minimising EMF exposure in the home and other places where members of the public spend much time.

The minimum action regarding RF and microwave EMF exposure should be:

- Strongly reinforce the current Department of Health guidance that children and young people under 16 years of age should only use a mobile phone when essential
- The DECT cordless phone standard should be changed so that they emit microwaves only when in use and not continuously
- The Department of Health should require that GPs gather information from patients who live near to mobile phone masts reporting ill-health problems. If possible, epidemiological and ecological studies that document levels of emissions and exposures should also be carried out
- Base station transmitters should not be located on lampposts close to homes, or on the walls of residential properties.

What is really concerning is that there may be no safe threshold level of man-made electric and magnetic fields across a wide range of frequencies. According to the late Neil Cherry, who was a Professor of Environmental Health at Lincoln University, New Zealand, the only safe exposure level is zero, a position confirmed by dose-response trends in epidemiological studies. He was a prolific researcher and writer on the science of EMFs and health (see Resources). Current health reports regarding adverse health effects of mobile phone base station radiation suggest that it would be advisable to keep RF signal strength levels in homes and schools below 0.05 volts per metre.

We repeat that, in our view, the evidence against EMF exposure and health is *far* more damning than that for the dangers of 'passive smoking'.

We accept that the jury is still out on many of the findings. Nevertheless, given the weight of existing evidence on power-frequency and mobile phone EMFS, we feel the time for precaution is now.

Endnotes

1   New York State Power Lines Project, Scientific Advisory Panel, *Biological Effects of Power Lines: Final Report*, New York State Department of Health, New York, NY, July 1987; Adey, W. R., *Evidence For Tissue Interactions With Microwave and Other Non-ionizing Electromagnetic Fields in Cancer Promotion*, First International Seminar, 'The Biophysics of Cancer', Charles University, Prague, July 1987; Smith, C.W. and Best, S., *Electromagnetic Man*, Dent, 1989.

2   Brodeur, Paul, *The Zapping of America*, Norton and Co., 1987, New York. Originally published in the New Yorker magazine.

3   Kane, R., *Cellular Telephone Russian Roulette*, Vantage Press, 2001; Carlo, G. and Schramm, M., *Cell Phones: Invisible hazards in a wireless age*. Caroll & Graff, 2001; Avalon Travel, 2003.

4   *Stewart (IEGMP) Report*, 2000, *Mobile Phones and Health*, ISBN 0 85951 450 1, available from the UK NRPB for £20. Also free at: www.iegmp.org.uk

5   *Stewart Report* update 2005, *Mobile Phones and Health*. Document of the NRPB Vol.15 No.5, 2004. Available at: www.hpa.org.uk/radiation

6   California report, a 560-page report. *An Evaluation of the Possible Risks From Electric and Magnetic Fields (EMFs) From Power Lines, Internal Wiring, Electrical Occupations and Appliances*, 2002. The report (with good references) is available at::
    http://www.dhs.ca.gov/ehib/emf/RiskEvaluation/riskeval.html An excellent summary and commentary on it by Professor Denis Henshaw of Bristol University is available at: www.electric-fields.bris.ac.uk/Careport.pdf

7   See: www.rkpartnership.co.uk/sage

8   Wertheimer, N. & Leeper, E., *Electrical Wiring Configurations and Childhood Cancer*, American Journal of Epidemiology, March 1979

9   *See reference number 7*

10 See: www.leukaemiaconference.org

11 Milham, S. & Ossiander, E. M., *Historical evidence that residential electrification caused the emergence of the childhood leukemia peak*, Medical Hypotheses Mar; 56(3):290-5, 2001

12 Davanipour, Z. et al, *Amyotrophic lateral sclerosis and occupational exposure to electromagnetic fields*, Bioelectromagnetics, 18(1):28-35, 1997

13 Foster, R. and Kreitzman, L., *Rhythms of Life*, Profile Books, 2004

14 *Microwave News*, 1 October 2005

15 1999 paper updated by Henshaw, D. L., 2002, *Does our electricity distri-bution system pose a serious risk to public health?* Medical Hypotheses Jul; 59(1):39-51; Henshaw, D. L. & Reiter, R. J., 2005, *Do magnetic fields cause increased risk of childhood leukaemia via melatonin disruption?* Bioelectromagnetics Suppl 7:S86-97, and World Health Organisation International EMF Project Workshop on Sensitivity of Children to EMF, June 2004, Istanbul, Turkey. See: www.who.int/peh-emf/meetings/archive/en/henshaw.pdf, and also: www.electric-fields.bris.ac.uk/melatoninpaper.pdf

16 Cardis, E. et al, *Risk of thyroid cancer after exposure to 131I in child-hood,* Journal of the National Cancer Institute, May 18; 97(10):724-32 and 703-5, 2005; Okeanov, A. E. et al, 2004 *National cancer registry to assess trends after the Chernobyl accident,* Swiss Medical Weekly, Oct 30; 134(43-44):645-9.

17 For information on EMFs and powerlines, see: www.emfs.info

18 *See reference number 17*

19 Sims S. & Dent P., 2005, *High-voltage overhead powerlines and property values: A residential study in the UK,* Urban Studies 42 (4), April

20 Eger, H. et al, *The influence of being physically near to a cell phone trans-mission mast on the incidence of cancer,* Umvelt–Medizin–Gesellschaft 17, 4, 2004

21 Oberfeld, G. et al, *The microwave syndrome – further aspects of a Spanish study,* Presented at 4th International Workshop on Biological Effects of Electromagnetic Fields, Kos, Greece, 4-8 October 2004

22 See reference number 4

23 Lai, H. et al, *Effects of low-level microwave irradiation on amphetamine hyperthermia are blockable by naloxone and classically conditionable* Psychopharmacology 88; 3:354-361, 1986

24 Salford, L. G. et al, *Nerve cell damage in mammalian brain after expo-sure to microwaves from GSM mobile phones.* Environmental Health Perspectives June; 111(7):881-3; discussion A408, 2003

25 http://www.bbc.co.uk/crime/support/mobilephone.shtml

26 Doll, R. & Peto, R., 1981, *The Causes of Cancer: Quantitative Estimates of Avoidable Risks of Cancer in the United States Today,* Oxford University Press.

27 FDA, *What are the Radiation Risks from CT scans?* See: http://www.fda.gov/cdrh/ct/risks.html, 2005

28 Brenner, D. J. et al, *Estimated risks of radiation-induced fatal cancer from pediatric CT,* AJR Am J Roentgenol, 176:289-296, 2001

29 Kallen et al, *Delivery Outcome among Physiotherapists in Sweden: is Non-ionizing Radiation a Fetal Hazard?* Archives of Environmental Health,

37(2):81-84, 1982; Larsen et al, *Gender specific reproductive outcome and exposure to high frequency electromagnetic radiation among physiotherapists,* Scand. J. Work Environ. Health, Vol.17, pp. 324-329, 1991; Ouellet-Hellstrom, R. & Stewart, W. F., *Miscarriages among Female Physical Therapists who report using radio- and microwave- frequency electromagnetic radiation,* American J. of Epidemiology, 138(10), pp. 775-86, 1993, plus reply in American J. of Epidemiology, 141(3), p. 274; Shields, N. et al, *Short-wave Diathermy and Pregnancy: What is the Evidence?* Advances in Physiotherapy, 5:1:2-14, 2003

30   Blackman, C. F. et al, *Influence of Electromagnetic Fields on the Efflux of Calcium Ions from Brain Tissue in Vitro: A Three-Model Analysis Consistent with the Frequency Response up to 510 Hz,* Bioelectromagnetics, 9:215-227, 1988

31   *Microwave News* first reported the Thériault et al work in November/December 1994 issue. A number of papers were published over the next five years; Miller, A. et al, *Leukemia following occupational exposure to 60 Hz electric and magnetic fields among Ontario electric utility workers,* Am.J.Epi,144:150-160, 15 July 1996

32   Nordstrom et al, *Reproductive hazards among workers at high voltage substations,* Bioelectromagnetics, 4(1):91-101, 1983

33   Li, D. K. et al, *A population-based prospective cohort study of personal exposure to magnetic fields during pregnancy and the risk of miscarriage,* Epidemiology, Jan; 13(1):9-20, 2002

34   *New Scientist,* Cellphone radiation 'trapped' in train carriages, reporting Hondou, T., 2 May 2002

35   Terahertz Bridge, *Terahertz radiation in biological research, investigation on diagnostics, and study on potential genotoxic effects,* EU Commission programme 'Quality of Life and Management of Living Resources', Key Action 4, 2004

36   Gandhi, O. P. et al, *Calculation of induced current densities for humans by magnetic fields from electronic article surveillance devices,* Phys. Med. Biol. 46 2759-2771, 2001

37   Herzog, P. & Rieger, C. T., *Risk of cancer from diagnostic X-rays, Lancet.* 2004 Jan 31; 363(9406):345-51, 2004

38   *See reference number 33*

39   *See reference number 24*

40   Johansson, O. et al., 1994, 'Skin changes in patients claiming to suffer from "screen dermatitis": a two-case open-field provocation study', Exp Dermatol; 3:234-238; Johansson, O. & Liu, P-Y, 1995, 'Electrosensitivity', 'electrosupersensitivity' and 'screen dermatitis': preliminary observations

from on-going studies in the human skin, In: Proceedings of the COST 244: Biomedical Effects of Electromagnetic Fields – Workshop on Electromagnetic Hypersensitivity (ed. D. Simunic), EU/EC (DG XIII), Brussels/Graz, pp. 52-57; Johansson, O. et al., 1996, A screening of skin changes, with special emphasis on neurochemical marker antibody evaluation, in patients claiming to suffer from screen dermatitis as compared to normal healthy controls, Exp Dermatol; 5:279-285; Johansson, O. et al., 1999, A case of extreme and general cutaneous light sensitivity in combination with so-called 'screen dermatitis' and 'electrosensitivity' – a successful rehabilitation after vitamin A treatment – a case report, J Aust Coll Nutr & Env Med; 18:13-16; Johansson et al., 2001, Cutaneous mast cells are altered in normal healthy volunteers sitting in front of ordinary TVs/PCs – results from open-field provocation experiments, J Cutan Pathol; 28:513-519; Johansson, O., 2002, Screen dermatitis and electrosensitivity: Preliminary observations in the human skin Proceedings of the conference 'Electromagnetic Environments and Health in Buildings', 16-17 May, at the Royal College of Physicians, London, U.K.

41   FSA, Project G10008, *Evaluating the risks associated with using GMOs in human foods,* Technical report, 2003 see: www.food.gov.uk/multimedia/pdfs/gmnewcastlereport.pdf

42   Schiff, M. 1995, *The Memory of Water,* Thorsons/HarperCollins

43   Irwin, M. R. et al, *Effects of a behavioral intervention, tai chi chih, on varicella-zoster virus specific immunity and health functioning in older adults,* Psychosomatic Medicine, 65:824-830, 2003

44   Leitgeb, N. & Schröttner, J., *Electro-sensibility and Electromagnetic Hypersensitivity,* Bioelectromagnetics, 24:387-394, 2003

45   Studies reviewed in Irvine, N., *Definition, Epidemiology and Management of Electrical Sensitivity,* UK Health Protection Agency – Radiation Protection Division, November 2005; Rubin, J., et al, *Electromagnetic Hypersensitivity: A Systematic Review of Provocation Studies,* Psychosomatic Medicine 67:224–232, 2005

46   Kimata, H., *Effect of Humor on Allergen-Induced Wheal Reactions,* Research letter, JAMA 285;738, 2001

47   Koskowski, *The Habit of Tobacco Smoking,* Staples Press, pp. 78-92, 1955

48   Wynder, E. & Graham, E., *Tobacco Smoking As A Possible Etiologic Factor in Bronchiogenic Carcinoma,* JAMA 143:329-336, 1950; Levin, M. L. et al, *Cancer and tobacco smoking,* JAMA 143:336-338, 1950

49   Doll, R. & Hill, A. B., *Smoking and carcinoma of the lung. Preliminary report,* BMJ ii:739-748, 1950

50   Doll, R. & Hill, A. B., *A study of the aetiology of carcinoma of the lung*, BMJ ii:1271-1286, 1952

51   EEA, *Late Lessons from Early Warnings: the precautionary principle 1896-2000*, European Environment Agency, ISBN 9291673234, 2001

52   Ibid

53   Hansard, UK Parliament, Lords Hansard, 210328w03, 28 March 2001.

54   Lipton, B., *The Biology of Belief*, Elite Books, 2005

55   Blackman, C. F. et al, *Influence of Electromagnetic Fields on the Efflux of Calcium Ions from Brain Tissue in Vitro: A Three-Model Analysis Consistent with the Frequency Response up to 510 Hz*, Bioelectromagnetics, 9:215-227, 1988; Blackman, C. F., *ELF effects on calcium homeostasis*, In *Extremely low frequency electromagnetic fields: The question of cancer*, Wilson, Stevens, Anderson Eds, Battelle Press, 187-208, 1990

56   Adey, W. R., *Cell and Molecular Biology Associated with Radiation Fields of Mobile Telephones*, in Review of Radio Science, 1996-1999, Stone & Ueno, eds. OUP, 845-872, 1999

57   Szent-Györgi, A., 1960, *Introduction to a Submolecular Biology*, Academic Press, New York

58   Weinhold, F., *A new twist on molecular shape*, Nature 411:539-541, 2001

59   *See reference number 54*

60   Doll, R. & Hill, A. B. *Lung cancer and other causes of death in relation to smoking. A second report on the mortality of British doctors*, BMJ, ii:1071, 1956

61   Milham, S., *Carcinogenicity of Electromagnetic Fields*, European Journal of Oncology, 3-2:93-100, 1998

62   *See reference number 11*

63   *See reference number 8*

64   *Microwave News, NCRP Draft Recommendations on EMF Exposure Guidelines,* /www.microwavenews.com/ncrp1.html, 1995

65   Polk, C. and Postow, E. (edited by), *Handbook of Biological Effects of Electromagnetic Fields,* CRC Press, 1996

66   Ahlbom, A. B. et al, *A pooled analysis of magnetic fields and childhood leukaemia*, British Journal of Cancer Sep; 83(5):692-8, 2000; Greenland, S. et al, *A pooled analysis of magnetic fields, wire codes and childhood leukaemia*. Epidemiology, 11:624-634, 2000; Wartenberg, D., *Residential EMF Exposure and Childhood Leukaemia: Meta-analysis and population attributable risk*, Bioelectromagnetics, Suppl. 5:S86-104, 2001

67   Kabuto, M. et al, *A case-control study of childhood leukemia and*

residential power-frequency magnetic fields, Int J Cancer (in print), 2004. Conference version available here:
http://www.leukaemiaconference.org/programme/posters/day3-kabuto.pdf

68 Ahlbom, A. B., *Childhood leukaemia and electromagnetic radiation – a review of epidemiological studies*, 2004 available at:
http://www.leukaemiaconference.org/programme/day3.asp

69 Draper, G. et al, *Childhood cancer in relation to distance from high voltage power lines in England and Wales: a case-control study*, BMJ, 330(7503):1290, 2005

70 Coleman, M. & Shah, A., in CHILDREN with LEUKAEMIA Conference Proceedings, 2004 available from:
http://www.leukaemiaconference.org/programme/day1.asp

71 IARC, *Static and Extremely Low-frequency (ELF) Electric and Magnetic Fields*, 2002, available from:
www-cie.iarc.fr/htdocs/monographs/vol80/80.html

72 NCI, US National Cancer Institute, please see:
http://seer.cancer.gov/publications/childhood/leukemia.pdf and:
www.cancer.gov/cancertopics/factsheet/NCI-childhood-cancers-research

73 Fews, A. P. et al, *Increased exposure to pollutant aerosols under high voltage power lines,* International Journal of Radiation Biology, 75(12), 1505-1521, 1999; Fews, A. P. et al, *Lung cancer risk estimate in people living near high voltage powerlines*, Presented at the 23rd Annual Bioelectromagnetics Meeting, 10-14 June, St Paul, Minnesota, 2001

74 *See reference number 69*

75 Coghill, R. et al, *ELF Electric and Magnetic fields in the bedplace of children with leukaemia: a case control study*, Eu.J.Can Prevent, v.5-3: 153-8, June 1996; Miller, A. et al, *Leukemia following occupational exposure to 60 Hz electric and magnetic fields among Ontario electric utility workers*, Am.J.Epi,144:150-160, 15 July 1996

76 *See reference number 6*

77 Lee, G. M. et al, *A nested case-control study of residential and personal magnetic field measures and miscarriages.* Epidemiology Jan; 13(1):21-31, 2002; Li D. K. et al, *A population-based prospective cohort study of personal exposure to magnetic fields during pregnancy and the risk of miscarriage,* Epidemiology Jan; 13(1):9-20, 2002

78 Perry, F. S., *Environmental power-frequency magnetic fields and suicide*, Health Physics, 41:267-277, 1981; Perry, F. S., *Power frequency magnetic field: depressive illness and myocardial infarction,* Public Health, 103:177-180, 1989; Savitz, D. A., *Prevalence of depression*

among electrical workers, American Journal of Industrial Medicine, 25:165-176, 1994

79   Sobel, E. et al, *Occupations with exposure to electromagnetic fields: a possible risk factor for Alzheimer's disease*, American Journal of Epidemiology, 142:515-524, 1995; Sobel, E. et al, *Elevated risk of Alzheimer's disease among workers with likely electromagnetic field exposure*, Neurology, Dec; 47(6):1477-81, 1996; Savitz, D. A. et al, *Magnetic field exposure and neurodegenerative disease mortality among electrical utility workers*, Epidemiology, 9:398-404, 1998c; Savitz, D. A. et al, *Electrical occupations and neuro-degenerative disease: analysis of U.S. mortality data*, Archives of Environmental Health Jan-Feb; 53(1):71-4, 1998b

80   Strickland, D. et al, *Amyotrophic lateral sclerosis and occupational history*, Arch Neurol 53:730-733, 1996; Johansen, C. & Olsen, J. H., *Mortality from amyotrophic lateral sclerosis and other chronic disorders and electric shocks among utility workers*, Am J Epi Aug 15;148(4):362-8, 1998; Savitz, D. A. et al, *Electrical occupations and neurodegenerative disease: analysis of US mortality data*, Arch Envir Health, 53:71-4, 1998b

81   Kundi, M., *Electromagnetic Fields and the Precautionary Principle*, in the Proceedings of the 2004 International Conference on the Causes of Childhood Leukaemia, CHILDREN with LEUKAEMIA Charity, available to be downloaded from: www.leukaemiaconference.org/programme/day5.asp

82   Sadcikova, M., *Clinical manifestations of reactions to microwave irradiation in various occupational groups*, in Biological Effects and Health Hazards of Microwave Radiation. WHO symposium, Polish Medical Publishers, 261-267, 1974

83   Silverman, C., *Epidemiologic Approach to the Study of Microwave Effects*, Bull. N.Y. Acad. Sci., 55-11:1166-118, 1979

84   McKinlay, A., *Possible health effects related to the use of radiotelephones*: Recommendations of a European Commission Expert Group, 1996

85   COST244bis (1998) Proceedings from Cost 244bis International Workshop on Electromagnetic Fields and Non-Specific Health ymptoms. 19-20 Sept 1998, Graz, Austria; and COST, 2000_244bis Working Group Report. DGXIII, E.C., Final Report 2003-11-03, EU. On EC website.

86   www.cost281.org

87   Leiss, W. & Paoli, *Risk Analysis: Facing the New Millennium*, Proceedings of 9th Annual Conference of Society for Risk Analysis, October 1999. For a fuller discussion of this perspective see chapter one in: Douglas Powell

& William Leiss, *Mad Cows and Mothers Milk: The Perils of Poor Risk Communication*, McGill-Queens University Press, 1997

88   WHO, 1998,
     www.who.int/docstore/peh-emf/publications/facts_press/efact/efs183.html

89   *Table compiled from the following and other sources:* Heynick & Polson,
     *Human Exposure to RF Radiation: A Comprehensive Review Pertinent to
     Air Force Operations.* Brooks Air Force Base, AL/OE-TR-1996-0035
     (earlier versions circulated), 1996; Durney, C.H.et al, *RF Radiation
     Dosimetry Handbook* (2nd Ed), USAF School of Aerospace Medicine, Brooks,
     A. F. B., TX, Report SAM-TR-78-22, 1978; Hankin, N. N., *RF Radiation:
     Environmental Exposure Levels and RF Radiation Emitting Sources*, U.S.
     EPA Technical Report EPA 520/1-85-014, 1985; Heynick, L. N., Critique
     of the Literature on Bioeffects of RF Radiation: A Comprehensive Review
     Pertinent to Air Force Operations, USAF School of Aerospace Medicine,
     Brooks Air Force Base, TX, Report USAFSAM-TR-87-3, 1987; Janes,
     D. E., *Radiation Surveys – Measurement of Leakage Emissions and
     Potential Exposure Fields*, Bulletin N.Y. Acad. Med., Vol. 55, No. 11,
     pp. 1021-1041, 1979; Janes, D. E., et al, *RF Radiation Levels in Urban
     Areas*, Radio Science, Vol. 12, No.6S, pp. 49-56, 1977; Tell, R. A. &
     Mantiply, E. D., *Population exposure to VHF and UHF broadcast
     radiation in the United States*, Proc. IEEE 68(1):6-12, 1980; Solon,
     L. R., *A local health agency approach to a permissible environmental
     level for microwave and radiofrequency radiation,* Bulletin NY Acad.
     Med. 55(11):1251-1266, 1979; Zaret, M. M., 1978, Nonionizing
     radiational injury of humans. In Congress Proceedings J Ninth
     International Congress of the French Society of Radio protection;
     Szmigielski, S. & Gil, J., *Electromagnetic fields and neoplasms*, In
     Electromagnetic Bio-interaction, Eds: Franceschetti et al, Plenum
     Press, NY, pp. 81-98, 1989; WHO, Environmental Health Criteria 16,
     ISBN 92 4 154076 1, 1981; *Stewart (IEGMP) Report, Mobile Phones
     and Health,* ISBN 0 85951 450 1, available from the UK NRPB for
     £20. Also free at: www.iegmp.org.uk

90   Trade & Industry Select Committee (UK Parliament) Minutes of 13 March
     2001 (27.03.2001), and 10th 2001 Report HC 330

91   REFLEX report, 2004, QLK4-CT-1999-01574/REFLEX/Final Report, avail-
     able at: http://www.verum-foundation.de

92   Lai, H., et al., *Microwave irradiation affects radial-arm maze performance
     in the rat*, Bioelectromagnetics 15:95-104, 1994; Wang & Lai, H., *Acute
     exposure to pulsed 2450-MHz microwaves affects water-maze perform-
     ance of rats.* Bioelectromagnetics, January, 21:52-56, 2000; Lai, H.,

Interaction of microwaves and a temporally incoherent magnetic field on spatial learning in the rat. Physiology & Behavior Oct 15;82(5):785-9, 2004

93 *See reference number 24*

94 See www.mwn.com

95 Frey, A. H., *Headaches from Cellular Telephones: Are they Real and What Are the Implications?* Environmental Health Perspectives 106(3):101-103, 1998

96 Leszczynski, D., et al. 2002. Effects of mobile phone radiation on gene and protein expression in vitro. Abstract 14-6. Bioelectromagnetics Society annual meeting, June, Quebec. http://www.bioelectromagnetics.org/doc/bems2002-abstracts.pdf

97 *Daily Telegraph*, 20 June 2002

98 Gandhi, O. P. et al, *Electromagnetic Absorption in the Human Head and Neck for Mobile Telephones*, IEEE Transactions on Microwave Theory and Techniques, 44, pp. 1884-1897, Oct 1996; Gandhi, O. P. & Kang, G., *Some Present Problems and a Proposed Experimental Phantom for SAR Compliance Testing of Cellular Telephones*, Physics in Medicine and Biology, 47, May 2002

99 see www.emfacts.com/papers/children_mobiles.pdf

100 Ibid

101 Edström, S., in Göteborgs-Posten, 13 December, 1999

102 Binhi, V., *Report from Russia – EMFs and Human Health*, 2003 http://www.emrnetwork.org/position/binhi_2_03.pdf

103 *Panorama*, BBC1, UK TV, 24 May 1999

104 Hardell, L. et al, Case-control study on radiology work, medical x-ray investigations, and use of cellular telephones as risk factors for brain tumors. Medscape General Medicine, May; 4;2(2):E2, 2000; Hardell, L. et al, Ionizing radiation, cellular telephones and the risk for brain tumours. European Journal of Cancer Prevention Dec; 10(6):523-9, 2001; Hardell, L. et al, Cellular and cordless telephones and the risk for brain tumours, European Journal of Cancer Prevention Aug; 11(4):377-86, 2002; Hardell, L. et al, Further aspects on cellular and cordless phones and brain tumours, International Journal of Oncology, 22:399-407, 2003; Hardell, L. et al, *Use of cellular telephones and brain tumour risk in urban and rural areas*, Occupational and Environmental Medicine, June; 62:390-394, 2005; Hardell, L. et al, *Pooled analysis of two case-control studies on the use of cellular and cordless telephones and the risk of benign brain tumours diagnosed during 1997-2003*, Int J Oncology 28:509-519, 2006; Lonn, S. et al, 2005, *Long term mobile*

phone use and brain tumour risk, American Journal of Epidemiology, 161:6, 526-535.

105 Hepworth, S. J., *Mobile phone use and risk of glioma in adults: case-control study,* BMJ online first, 20 January 2006; Schoemaker, M. J. et al, *Mobile phone use and risk of acoustic neuroma: results of the Interphone case-control study in five North European countries,* Br.J.Cancer, September 2005 www.nature.com/bjc/journal/vaop/ncurrent/abs/6602764a.html; Schüz, J., *Cellular Phones, Cordless Phones, and the Risks of Glioma and Meningioma,* A.J.E. Advance January 2006

106 Von Klitzing, L., *Low-Frequency pulsed electromagnetic fields influence EEG of man,* Physica Medica 11:77-80, 1995; Mann, K. & Roschke, J., *Effects of pulsed high-frequency electromagnetic fields on human sleep,* Neuropsychobiology 33:41-47, 1996; Krause, C. M. et al, *Effects of electromagnetic field emitted by a cellular phone on the EEG during a memory task.* Neuroreport 20 March: 11(4) 761-4, 2000

107 Borbely, A. et al, *Pulsed high-frequency electromagnetic field affects human sleep and sleep electroencephalogram.* Neuroscience letters, 275 (3):207-210, 1999; Huber, R. et al, *Electromagnetic fields, such as those from mobile phones, alter regional cerebral blood flow and sleep and waking EEG,* J Sleep Res 11:280-295, 2002

108 Loughran, S. P. et al, *The effect of electromagnetic fields emitted by mobile phones on human sleep.* NeuroReport. Nov 28;16(17):1973-6., 2005

109 Tice, R. R. et al, *Genotoxicity of radiofrequency signals. I. Investigation of DNA damage and micronuclei induction in cultured human blood cells.* Bioelectromagnetics 23:113-126, 2002

110 Pedersen, G.F. & Andersen, J.B, 1999, *RF and ELF Exposure from Cellular Phone Handsets: TDMA and CDMA systems,* Rad.Prot.Dos.83, 1-2, 131-138

111 Szmigielski, S., *Cancer morbidity in subjects occupationally exposed to high frequency (RF & microwave) electromagnetic radiation,* The Science of the Total Environment 180:9-18, 1996

112 Garber, K., *Lymphoma rate rise continues to baffle researchers,* J. National Cancer Institute, 93(7):494-496, 2001

113 Hocking, B. et al, *Cancer Incidence and mortality and proximity to TV towers,* Medical Journal of Australia, vol 165(2):601-605, December 1996

114 Hocking, B. et al, *Decreased survival for childhood leukemia in proximity to TV towers,* Annual Scientific Meeting of the Royal Australasian College of Physicians in Adelaide 2-5 May 2000

115 Dolk, H. et al, *Cancer Incidence near Radio & TV Transmitters in Great*

Britain, American Journal of Epidemiology, 145; 1:1-9 (Part 1) and 10-17 (Part 2), 1997

116 Naila Study, *The Influence of Being Physically Near to a Cell Phone Transmission Mast on the Incidence of Cancer,* Umwelt-Medizin-Gesellschaft 17,4, 2004. Available at: http://www.powerwatch.org.uk/news/20041118_naila.pdf

117 Wolf, R. & D., *Increased Incidence of cancer near a cellphone transmitter station,* International Journal of Cancer Prevention 1(2):123-128, 2004 (*available at www.powerwatch.org.uk*)

118 Abelin, T. et al, *Study of health effects of the Shortwave Transmitter Station of Schwarzenburg, Berne, Switzerland,* Univ. Berne, Inst. for Social and Preventative Medicine, Bundesamt für Energiewirtschaft Schriftenreihe Studie 56, 1995

119 Kolodynski, A. & Kolodynska, V., *Motor and psychological functions of school children living in the area of the Skrunda Radio Location Station in Latvia,* The Science of the Total Environment 180:88-93, Elsevier, 1996

120 Navarro, E. A. et al, *The Microwave Syndrome: A Preliminary Study in Spain,* Electromagnetic Biology and Medicine, 22; 2:161-179, 2003

121 *See reference number 21*

122 Santini, R. et al, *Study of the health of people living in the vicinity of mobile phone base stations,* Pathologie Biologie (Paris); 50:369-373, 2002

123 Zwamborn, A. P. M. et al, *Effects of Global Communication system radio-frequency fields on Well Being and Cognitive Functions of human subjects with and without subjective complaints,* 2003. The report is available at: www.ez.nl/beleid/home_ond/gsm/docs/TNO-FEL_REPORT_03148_Definitief.pdf

124 Gallerano, G. P., *Terahertz radiation in Biological Research – Investigations on Diagnostics and study on potential Genotoxic Effects,* THz-BRIDGE, ENEA QLK4-CT-2000-00129, 2004

125 ICNIRP, *Epidemiology of Health Effects of Radiofrequency Exposure,* Environmental Health Perspectives 112:17, 1741-1754, 2004 www.icnirp.de/documents/epiRFreviewPublishedinEHPDec04.pdf

126 NRPB, *Review of the Scientific Evidence for Limiting Exposure to Electromagnetic Fields (0–300 GHz),* Documents of the NRPB:15-3, 2004a. Available from: www.hpa.org.uk/radiation

127 *See reference number 5*

128 *See reference number 4*

129 WHO, 2005, website: http://www.who.int/peh-emf/en/

Note: an extended list of these references is available on the Powerwatch website, listed in order of the first author of each paper.

Resources

Organisations

CHILDREN with LEUKAEMIA

Only about 2 per cent of the total research spend on all cancers goes on investigating ways of preventing them. All the author royalties from the sale of this book are being donated to CHILDREN with LEUKAEMIA, the UK charity that *does* investigate the causes of leukaemia and related child cancers so that future families will not have to face the devastating consequences of this dreadful illness. You can get further information about the charity from their main website www.leukaemia.org or call them, in London, on 0207 404 0808.

You can find details of their five-day 2004 International Scientific Conference on the possible causes of child cancer, complete with all presentations, at www.leukaemiaconference.org.

Powerwatch

Alasdair and Jean Philips run Powerwatch, an independent organisation devoted to disseminating research and information on EMFs. The background is given on our website, www.powerwatch.org.uk, where we also have a 'news' service. You can become a subscriber to the website and be kept up to date with the latest thinking, articles of specific interest and reports on EMFs. Powerwatch has published a number of books on the subject of EMFs (see Futher Reading). These can be purchased from the EMFields website at www.emfields.org/publications/overview.asp.

Scientific instrument hire

Alasdair Philips designs scientific instruments for measuring EMFs. See the www.emfields.org website, or telephone 01353 778814 for details. The instruments are easy to use even if you are not scientifically trained or qualified, and come with simple instructions. They allow you to compare the readings you get with the international research recommendations for good health.

The instruments include:

- Powerfrequency meters to measure fields from powerlines, substations, cables, house wiring, electrical appliances, exposures in vehicles and public areas.
- Radiofrequency meters to measure the microwave radiation from mobile phone masts, radar, mobile and cordless phones, wireless networked computers, baby monitors and burglar alarms, exposures in vehicles and public places.
- Negative air ionisers to improve the quality of the environment in which you live and work.

Alasdair Philips continues to develop new instruments as better techniques of affordable measurement become available.

EMFields, the mail order service affiliated to Powerwatch, sells and hires the instruments described above, and also advises on, and sells, fully tested ways of screening microwave radiation coming into the house from mobile phone masts and other sources of microwave radiation. It offers an increasing range of personal protection for those people who experience health effects from such transmitting equipment. See www.emfields.org

Websites

Powerwatch maintains an up-to-date list of what we regard as the most useful websites. Most of these have links to other relevant sites. We recommend that you start with www.powerwatch.org.uk/gen/resource.asp: here you'll find links to all the big official sites, campaigns, general information and so on. We've also included a selection below.

For general, non-official information on EMFs
Powerwatch – www.powerwatch.org.uk
Microwave News (all types of EMF) – www.microwavenews.com
Neil Cherry's papers – www.neilcherry.com
EMF news resource – www.buergerwelle.de/english_start.html
EM Hazard and Therapy Newsletter –
  www.em-hazardtherapy.com
Ionising radiation in the environment – www.llrc.org
Don Maisch's excellent site (Tasmania) – www.emfacts.com
USA EMF-Guru site – www.emfguru.org
James Beal's site – www.emfinterface.com
EMF Safety Superstore – www.lessemf.com/emf-shie.html
EMR Association of Australia – www.emraa.org.au
EMR Network USA – www.emrnetwork.org

Foresight Preconception care –
  www.foresight-preconception.org.uk
Magnets and EMF information – www.cogreslab.co.uk
Green Clay – www.wholistichealthdirect.co.uk

UK masts and mobile phones
EMR research Registered Charity – www.radiationresearch.org
Mast Action – www.mastaction.co.uk
Mast Sanity – www.mastsanity.org
TETRAwatch – www.tetrawatch.net
UK phone masts – www.sitefinder.radio.gov.uk or
www.starweave.com

Powerlines
Bristol University – www.electric-fields.bris.ac.uk
SAGE – www.rkpartnership.co.uk/sage/
National Grid EMF information – www.emfs.info/default.asp
REVOLT – www.revolt.co.uk
Trentham Environmental Action – www.revolt.co.uk/trentham

Electrical Hypersensitivity
Electrosensitivity UK (charity) – www.electrosensitivity.org.uk
Swedish site on EHS (in English) – www.feb.se
GreenHealthWatch – www.ehn.clara.net/
Low-EMF phones – www.teloray.se

UK practitioners specialising in EMFs

Doctors
The doctors listed below have specialist knowledge of electrical
  hypersensitivity (EHS). Note that they work in private prac-
  tice, not the NHS.
Dr David Dowson, 01225 475 508 (Bath and London)
Dr Jean Monro, 01442 261333 (Hemel Hempstead)
Dr Monro is Medical Director of The Breakspear (private day)

Hospital. She specialises in the treatment of allergies and environmental illness.

Surveyors

John Meredith, chartered surveyor, 0207 341 4333 (London and the South East)

Seraph Surveying Services, Colin Gell, 0115 962 2888
Specialises in wayleaves and easements

Electromagnetic and geopathic energy surveyor

Roy Riggs, 01273 732523, www.royriggs.co.uk

Further reading

Books

Beck, M., *The Joy Diet*, Piatkus, 2003

Becker, Robert O. (MD), & Andrew A. Marino, *Electromagnetism and Life*, SUNY Press, Albany, NY, 1982

Becker, Robert O. (MD), & Gary Seldon, *The Body Electric: Electromagnetism and the Foundation of Life*, William Morrow and Company, Inc., New York, 1985

Becker, Robert O., *Cross Currents – The Perils of Electropollution, The Promise of Electromedicine*, Tarcher, 1991. An excellent overview.

Brodeur, P., *Currents of Death*, Simon & Schuster, 1989. A brilliant background read, originally published in the *New Yorker*.

Brodeur, Paul, *The Great Power-Line Cover-Up: How the Utilities and the Government Are Trying to Hide the Cancer Hazards Posed by Electromagnetic Fields*, Little, Brown and Company, Boston, Mass., 1993

Brodeur, Paul, *The Zapping of America*, Norton and Co., New York, 1987, Originally published in the *New Yorker* magazine.

Buckley, Dr S. J., *Gentle Birth, Gentle Mothering: The wisdom and science of gentle choices in pregnancy, birth and parenting*, 2005. See: http://sarahjbuckley.com

Campbell, D., *The Mozart Effect,* Hodder & Stoughton, 1997

Carlo, G. and Schramm, M., *Cell Phones: Invisible hazards in a wireless age*, Caroll & Graff, 2001; Avalon Travel, 2003. A top 'industry scientific insider' tells tales of 'dirty dealings' by the cell phone industry to make sure health fears are dismissed.

Clements-Croombe, D. (Ed.), *Electromagnetic Environments and Health in Buildings,* Spon Press, 2004. Good academic treatment.

Foster, R. and Kreitzman, L., *Rhythms of Life*, Profile Books, 2004. The science in some chapters is quite complex, but still a brilliant read.

Grant, L., *The Electrical Sensitivity Handbook – How EMFs are making people sick*, Weldon Publishing, 1995

Kane, R., *Cellular Telephone Russian Roulette,* Vantage Press, 2001. An insider's view of hidden cellular industry health issues.

Levitt, B. (Ed.) *Cell Towers: Wireless convenience? Or environmental hazard?* Safe Goods Publishing, 2001. An invaluable resource book, covering the presentations of the Cell Towers Forum, with chapters by many leading researchers and figures in the field.

Lipton B, *The Biology of Belief*, Elite Books, 2005

Nordstrom, G., *The Invisible Disease*, O Books, 2004. A book about EHS, mainly in Scandinavia.

Oschman, J. L., *Energy Medicine: The Scientific Basis*, Churchill Livingstone, 2000

Philips, A., & J., *Buying an EMF Safe Property*, available from EMFields

Philips, A., & J., *EMF and Microwave Protection for You and Your Family*, Available from EMFields

Philips, A., & J., *Mobile Phones and Masts, The Health Risks*, available from EMFields

Philips, A., & J., *Hypersensitivity, A Modern Illness,* available from EMFields

Philips, A., & J., *Influence of High-Frequency Electromagnetic Radiation at Non-Thermal Intensities on the Human Body* (a review of work by Russian and Ukranian researchers), available from EMFields

Polk, C., & Postow, E. (Eds.), *Biological Effects of Electromagnetic Fields*, 2nd Ed, Ch.7, 275-294, CRC Press, 1996

Reiter, R. J. and Robinson, J., *Melatonin,* Bantam, 1996. Good general-purpose book about the importance of melatonin.

Royal College of Physicians, *Allergy: The unmet need*, 2003

Saunders, T., *The Boiled Frog Syndrome*, Wiley-Acadamy, 2002. An excellent guide to our slow environmental poisoning.

Schiff, M, *The Memory of Water*, Thorsons/HarperCollins, 1995

Smith, C., W. and Best, S., *Electromagnetic Man*, Dent, 1989. An old, but very good, introduction. Now out of print, you will need to order it at your local library.

Wolverton, B. C., *Eco-Friendly House Plants*, Weidenfeld & Nicolson, 1996

Index